D0066691

WHAT YOU CAN
WHEN YOU CAN

··

HEALTHY LIVING ON *Your* TERMS

CARLA BIRNBERG & RONI NOONE

SEAL PRESS

What You Can When You Can

Copyright © 2015 Carla Birnberg and Roni Noone

All rights reserved. No part of this book may be reproduced or transmitted in any form without written permission from the publisher, except by reviewers who may quote brief excerpts in connection with a review.

Library of Congress Cataloging-in-Publication Data

Birnberg, Carla.
What you can when you can : Healthy living on your terms / Carla Birnberg and Roni Noone.
pages cm
ISBN 978-1-58005-573-4
1. Women—Health and hygiene. 2. Women—Psychology. 3. Motivation (Psychology) 4. Health. I. Noone, Roni. II. Title.
RA778.N785 2015
613—dc23
2014035547

Published by
Seal Press
A Member of the Perseus Books Group
1700 Fourth Street
Berkeley, California
Sealpress.com

Interior design by Domini Dragoone
Author photos on page 161 (left, Carla Birnberg) © Nathan Hall; (right, Roni Noone) © Lee Morton www.clickspark.it
Printed in the United States of America
Distributed by Publishers Group West

THIS BOOK IS DEDICATED TO OUR BLOG READERS.
The folks who read those early, barely coherent posts and waited
patiently for us to find our voices. The people who watched our
interminable videos on YouTube, bad quality and all. Those who
responded to our tweets when we had no clue what a hashtag was.
And all our friends on Facebook we have yet to meet in person.

Whether you lurk or comment prolifically,
please know we appreciate you.

This book isn't just *for* you, it's *because* of you.

CONTENTS

PART IV: FOOD FOR THOUGHT

PART V: TRICKS OF THE TRADE

PART VI: BEFORE WE LET YOU GO

INTRODUCTION

• •

WE'RE ALL AWARE WE SHOULD EAT BETTER, exercise more, get better-quality rest, and so on. Tell us something we don't know, right? After all, every statistic we have about Americans and our health proves that, no matter how good our intentions are, we are failing to change the habits that undermine our well-being. So how do we achieve our healthy living goals when they're so daunting? Who has the time, the willpower, the resources to do all that nutritious eating, muscle building, and work-life balancing?

You do, actually. And we do too.

This is our story. This is your story. We know you. We *are* you.

How so? you might be asking. Let us tell you.

In this fast-paced world of ours, we know it can often seem like everything is all or nothing: if we're not skinny, we're fat; or if we're not cardio queens, we're lazy slobs; or if we're not perfect, we've failed.

Now, early on in this book we alert you to one of our primary messages: perfect is not coming. Accept that. But, even if we do accept that *and* we want to lose a few pounds or improve our cholesterol levels, that same all-or-nothing mentality can take over. We too easily

The WYCWYC way isn't about changing your life overnight: it's about knowing that the road to improvement is paved brick by brick, step by step, and by simply doing What You Can When You Can.

•••••••••●•••••••••

slide into thinking lifestyle changes need to happen all at once or they're not worth attempting at all. We've both done it.

For example, we've both gone down the path of completely over-hauling our diets and exercise routines, only to stick with it for a day or three or—okay, let's be completely honest—an hour.

> "I know! I'll food prep for the week on Sundays; we'll eat healthily all week. Oh! Oh! I'll sign up for yoga and go every day after work! Tomorrow I'll start running. Tomorrow. Tomorrow."

If you're anything like us, you end up not doing any Sunday food preparation and you don't even drive *past* the yoga class—because you have less than the "perfect" amount of time available.

> "Well, so much for that healthy eating plan; I can't even get to the store, let alone cook all Sunday. Yoga every day after work, HA! I'm lucky to make it through rush-hour traffic. And running? Yeah, Okay, I can't even find my shoes in the morning."

Sound familiar? You are definitely *not* alone.

After years of struggling to make changes in our lives—everything from diet to fitness to relationships—we figured out a not-so-secret secret that has helped us finally reach the goals we've struggled with for so long.

That secret: do WHAT YOU CAN WHEN YOU CAN.

Also known as WYCWYC. We pronounce it *wick-wick*.

Born from our longing to end perfectionist tendencies and stop the "start tomorrow" mindset, the WYCWYC mantra reminds us that doing WHAT WE CAN WHEN WE CAN is enough.

There is no "Tomorrow, I'm starting over."

There is no magic "best" day of the week.

There is no "this day is shot" because things didn't go as planned.

By doing what we can when we can, we—Carla and Roni—will reach (and have been reaching) our goals—this book being one of them.

While WYCWYC stands for "what you can when you can," it encapsulates so much more. WYCWYC is about acknowledging that doing your best—and making compromises when needed—is *always* enough.

"I missed my step class but that's okay; I'll take a walk with the family after dinner."

It's about seeking out every opportunity that interests you without feeling guilty or disappointed in yourself for not being perfect.

"Busiest day ever traveling for business. Too cold to walk. Jumped on the hotel 'dreadmill' instead."

It's even about balancing your current desires while *still* working toward your future goals.

"I really wanted fried mozzarella, so I ordered a soup for my entrée, skipped dessert, and drank sparkling water instead of wine."

WYCWYC is an approach to life that helps us break out of the negative cycles holding us back.

WHO IS THIS BOOK FOR?

This book is for everyone who is struggling with a sense of what we "should" do.

People who make New Year's resolutions to get healthy and then break them in the first week of the year.

People who find the *perfect* diet and stick to it completely—that is, until the next birthday party at work.

People paralyzed by a never-ending to-do list, buried under the clutter of life.

Maybe that's not exactly you. Bottom line, if you've ever questioned if doing the best you can is enough, then this book is for you.

If you've again and again promised yourself you'd make big changes, only to feel like a failure for never making progress, then this book is for you.

If you feel alone working toward your healthy-living goals and seek support and community, then this book is for you.

What you hold in your hands is a spark, a mantra, a state of mind.

WYCWYC is for anyone looking to break out of the negative, self-defeating cycles that prevent us from reaching our goals, whatever those goals may be.

HOW TO USE THIS BOOK

As you can probably tell, this book is *not* about "losing ten pounds by Friday so you can fit into that dress." We're done playing those games with our bodies and our minds.

This book is also not an eat-this-don't-eat-that guide, or a thirty-days-to-a-new-you plan.

In a way this book isn't even a book. The word "book" implies there's a beginning and an end. There is no end. This is a living, breathing thing—and, thanks to social media, it's also a vibrant online community. It's a way of life. It's a movement.

What you hold in your hands is simply inspiration. A few sparks. We want this book to be your launching pad. We want it to change the way you think about healthy living and goals.

To that end, we've organized *What You Can When You Can* into six parts. Though we include items to do throughout, we start out focusing on perspective with Part I: It's All About Mindset. In Part II, we guide you in how to Rethink and Take Charge. Since by Part III we're well into action territory, we provide many Daily Considerations of the WYCWYC approach. After that, we've grouped all the food-inspired chapters into Part IV: Food for Thought. By Part V, you'll be a pretty seasoned WYCWYCer, so there you'll find our many Tricks of the Trade. And in Part VI: Before We Let You Go, we wrap up with a few last-but-not-least chapters of final thoughts.

But the fun doesn't even end there, because in the back you'll find information about the wonderful world of social media, including sample WYCWYC nuggets to share with the community.

So, again, this journey is about starting to see just how many opportunities there are in every day to do WHAT YOU CAN WHEN YOU CAN in pursuit of your goals. We'd like this book to serve as your guide in doing just that. We hope you'll spend some time with it now, for inspiration, and then revisit it every time you feel overwhelmed or defeated. Use it to focus; use it to refocus. Use it to find motivation in the mundane.

Remember: it's not about starting over perfectly tomorrow. It's about doing WHAT YOU CAN WHEN YOU CAN today.

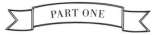

PART ONE

IT'S ALL ABOUT
MINDSET

JOIN A MOVEMENT

• •

OUR FIRST TIP MAY SEEM A LITTLE LOFTY, BUT hear us out.

WHAT YOU CAN WHEN YOU CAN is a movement. It's about being part of a community, and we know from experience how powerfully it works. We invite you to join us!

Reaching for challenges solo is never as effective as reaching out to others for their support, input, guidance, wisdom, encouragement, and shared enthusiasm. With all this, we can overcome pitfalls and get back on our healthier path.

This is where harnessing the power of WHAT YOU CAN WHEN YOU CAN comes in. It's easy—here's what you do.

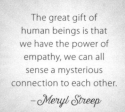

The great gift of human beings is that we have the power of empathy, we can all sense a mysterious connection to each other.

–Meryl Streep

#wycwyc

From Twitter to Facebook, Instagram to Tumblr to Pinterest, find a social media channel (or three) that matches your personality and communication style. You may discover, as we did, that you're drawn to different social media platforms at different times and for different

No one is an island.
True momentum is sparked and
maintained when we locate our
community and have a safe place
to share both our victories
and our struggles.

·············●●●·············

reasons. It doesn't matter where you post, or what device you use to do it—the key to WYCWYC is to know *you are not alone.*

The more you reach out and interact, the stronger your community becomes, and the stronger you become.

And for those of you new to social media—welcome to the wonderful world of online friendship!

It's okay if you're skeptical—just give it a try. At first it may feel like you've arrived solo at a cocktail party where everyone already knows each other; it feels that way to all of us. But the more you tweet, Instagram, Facebook, and Pin—using the hashtag #wycwyc—the more you'll see how encouraging and inspiring a positive community can be. (Check out Appendix A for some quick tips and a brief introduction to social media.)

Plus, you already have two friends waiting for you! Find us, Carla and Roni, at www.wycwyc.com, because we can't wait to meet you.

Online you will meet like-minded people who are also striving toward healthier living. In the WYCWYC community there are hundreds of other people who are

★ Making their own commitments

★ Celebrating their successes

* Struggling with a moment (or a month) of feeling stuck and stagnant, and turning to #wycwyc to get back on track

* Engaging and inspiring each other to make healthy changes

So, whether you share a victory or seek encouragement, with every post you'll generate a ripple effect in the WYCWYC movement. And it's because of this community that we succeeded in reaching our own healthy-living goals: because we had somewhere to turn when we needed inspiration to lift us toward new and higher goals.

What are you waiting for? Come join us!

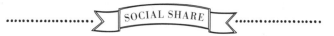

SOCIAL SHARE

Introduce yourself to the online community of WYCWYCers. Via Twitter, Facebook, Instagram, Pinterest, Tumblr, or the www.wycwyc.com blog use the #wycwyc hashtag so we can find you—share with us your healthy-living aspirations. #wycwyc

ACCEPT THAT PERFECT IS NEVER COMING

•••

WE'RE HERE TO LET YOU IN ON A LITTLE secret. Perfect is never coming. You will never be perfect. Your life will never be perfect.

We have another secret—it's *good* that you will never be perfect. None of us will. So what's the point of wasting time, energy, money, sweat, and tears on something that will never happen—on an unachievable ideal?

> I don't believe in perfection. I don't think there is such a thing. But the energy of wanting things to be great is a perfectionist energy.
>
> – *Reese Witherspoon*
>
> #wycwyc

"Perfect" is just a figment of human imagination. It's also a nasty distraction, one that obscures reality, making our dreams that much harder to achieve.

Coming to terms with the fact that "perfect" is an illusion opens the world to us, and helps us to achieve what is actually within reach, in *this* life, on *this* planet.

Life is imperfection. And, because of that, it helps to learn to accept imperfection—as well as how not to let whatever life throws at us derail us from our goals.

Once the notion of perfectionism is abolished, persistence is allowed its rightful place in guiding us in achieving our goals.

••••••••●●••••••••••

For example, let's say you've committed to walk for thirty minutes a day, but today you had to stay late at work, or run a last-minute errand, or *geesh*, a tire blew out on the way home. So now you've got only ten minutes for that walk.

Not at all ideal, and nowhere near perfect. Okay—but what do you do? Do you take a ten-minute walk? Or do you let this minor setback abort your goal?

Here's another scenario: You've decided to improve your diet— you're avoiding processed sugar and flour. But a coworker brings her famous homemade cookies to the office to celebrate a successful project. You eat one to share in the revelry, then another, and another.

What happens next? Do you stick to your plan for getting a salad at lunchtime, or do you grab a slice of pizza and decide tomorrow will be your new "start eating cleaner" day?

When we seek perfection, we fail. We cannot but fail, because perfection doesn't exist. Every day brings a new host of unexpected challenges and temptations that can derail us from our best intentions. The thing is, why should we berate ourselves for not being something it's impossible to be? It's when we learn to let go of idealized standards that we can finally step out of our own way and allow persistence to take over.

Yes, persistence.

Persistence keeps us moving, trying, striving—sticking to our goal and finding workable detours around the obstacles that will inevitably challenge our best-laid plans.

So let's revisit the scenarios mentioned above and consider WHAT YOU CAN do in each situation.

WHAT HAPPENED:
A delay at the dry cleaners cut twenty minutes out of your only exercise time for the day.

WHAT YOU CAN DO ABOUT IT:
Enlist the family in a jumping jacks contest to see who can last a full ten minutes.

WHAT HAPPENED:
You may have overindulged in the cookie department at that impromptu office celebration this morning.

WHAT YOU CAN DO ABOUT IT:
Consider them your dessert "points" for the next day or two— without feeling bad about it.

Persistence leaves room for success, even in the face of over-booked schedules and home-baked cookies, allowing us to take pride in what we achieved despite the challenges instead of crying over where we've fallen short.

We're inclined to trust Voltaire in thinking perfect is the enemy of good—especially since the desire for healthier and happier lives is very, very good. In fact, it's glorious! We encourage you to persist in your efforts; it's in those efforts that you will see glorious results.

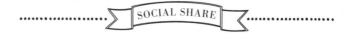

Try not to fear the flaws: flaws are part of being human. Instead, share them. Inspire others by sharing a way you've recently overcome the pursuit of perfection. #wycwyc

∞

HARNESS THE POWER OF BABY STEPS

● ●

LET'S THINK FOR A MOMENT ABOUT THE PHRASE
"baby steps." What are they?

Whether or not you're a parent, "baby steps" brings to mind a visual of tiny tentative moves forward— typically celebrated with great fanfare and photos, even when they end with a *plop* back down on the bahootie.

Part of why we recognize the tremendous effort these little shuffles take is that they signal progress—but there's more to it than that. They're also leaps of faith. We can imagine how scary it must feel to break from the secure routine of crawling

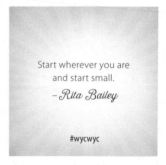

Start wherever you are
and start small.

– *Rita Bailey*

#wycwyc

in order to brave balancing on two legs. It's hard! That's why no baby has ever yanked herself to her feet, walked without wobbling, and soon thereafter run like a gazelle.

Instead, she stands, steps, falls, and tries again—over and over again. And we celebrate that persistence.

When we take baby steps toward doing What We Can When We Can every day, we set ourselves up for success in living healthy lives.

••••••••••●••••••••••

We're here to remind you that the baby steps toward healthy living are no different, and they shouldn't be celebrated any less. The seemingly small forward steps you may take today—"Let's make a healthy dinner tonight"—aren't any less significant than that baby's first efforts to grow and progress. And just as her accumulated efforts to walk eventually pay off, your own accumulated efforts, the tiny moves you can make tomorrow—"I'll take the stairs at work"—and the day after, and the day after that, all add up to create vast change over time.

Now, reaching this success will require squashing the urge to try for bigger and better too fast. Sure, we'd rather leap than toddle, and the resolution to make big changes quickly can be exciting, but experience has likely shown all of us that that approach rarely works. After a few days we find ourselves too sore, too tired, too burned-out—and we quit.

Whereas, by taking small steps in the right direction, day after day, we're far more likely to both gain and maintain a forward momentum. And we're here to tell you that small and steady *works*.

By refusing to set grandiose goals—"I'll go to the gym every day this week!"—and instead taking a more measured WYCWYC approach—"I'll work out once this week and twice next week"—we set ourselves up for a lasting success. This works in part because setting and achieving reachable goals creates the enthusiasm necessary to continue.

So, what might those goals be? Let's examine a few.

WHAT YOU WANT:

Let's say you want to join your coworkers in a 5K walk, but you pretty much never exercise and don't think you could finish. How might you go about achieving that goal?

WHAT YOU CAN DO TO GET IT:

Start by walking for five minutes before work and five minutes after. There's ten minutes of movement you weren't getting before, and it's not so hard to accomplish. Then keep at it, and keep adding—add a few minutes to each walking session as the weeks go by. In time, that 5K will be within reach, as will a glorious day with your friends.

WHAT YOU WANT:

You've decided you want to cut down on soda and drink more water, but it's tough—you love those bubbles!

WHAT YOU CAN DO TO GET IT:

Instead of quitting cold turkey, pour yourself a full glass of water alongside every soft drink. As time passes and you're drinking more water, slowly reduce the amount of soda you take in. Eventually, water will be your mainstay, and soda will be your special treat.

WHAT YOU WANT:

Your doctor told you increased muscle strength will reduce your back pain, but all those hyperfit women who go to the gym every morning intimidate you. How can you ever be like them?

WHAT YOU CAN DO TO GET IT:

The answer is, you don't try to be like them. You be yourself—and you start by checking out the website of the gym you've had your eye on. Next, just make an appointment to tour the facility. That's all. Then maybe buy a day pass, to take one of their classes and try out the Jacuzzi . . .

And pat yourself on the back for each single step you take toward your goal.

Overarching goals can feel overwhelming when we try to peer at the finish line from all the way back at the starting line. So, instead, set your sights on the step right in front of you. And when you've decided it's time to take that first step, do WHAT YOU CAN WHEN YOU CAN, and then do it again, consistently over time.

Crawl first.

Walk next.

Run someday.

And celebrate every step of the way.

> SOCIAL SHARE <

Take a baby step today—and snap a photo of yourself doing it. Then share your "selfie" online using the #wycwyc hashtag, and challenge others to guess what healthy habit you're working toward! #wycwyc

BE CONSISTENTLY FLEXIBLE

• •

WE DISCUSSED EARLIER HOW PERSISTENCE CAN help us attain our goals. Part of what makes persistence so effective is consistency—sticking to our goal day in, day out.

The challenge, however, comes when life conspires to derail our consistency.

You know what we're talking about. Let's say you're in a groove. You (finally) configured a routine that fits your schedule, allowing you to exercise, eat well, get enough sleep, and stay on track with your healthy living goals.

> We are what we repeatedly do. Excellence, then, is not an act, but a habit.
> – *Will Durant*,
> author of *The Story of Philosophy: The Lives and Opinions of the World's Greatest Philosophers*
> #wycwyc

It works well for you.

It's what you do.

Consistently.

For months now. Until . . . suddenly you're forced to abandon that consistency. Something comes up—a school vacation, a work deadline, even a sick family member—and you lose your routine.

It happens to all of us. The trouble is, once we get knocked off the conveyor belt—or treadmill—it can be hard to get back on again. It's also at times like this that our inner perfectionist can sneak back in to tell us we might as well give up.

But living the WYCWYC way is better than seeking perfection—which, you'll recall, we've already determined is unattainable. WYCWYC is about being consistent, and in an achievable, *flexible* way. We don't need to feel guilty about those cookies we had this morning. We can focus instead on getting right back on track for the meals and snacks to come.

Being consistent requires flexibility for the mere fact that life happens. For example, let's imagine . . .

WHAT HAPPENED:
A snow delay forced you to miss your spin class.

WHAT YOU CAN DO ABOUT IT:
Bundle up and take a walk around the office park at lunch.

WHAT HAPPENED:
You're facing a week of dinners out instead of healthy meals at home.

WHAT YOU CAN DO ABOUT IT:
Do WHAT YOU CAN with the menu, opting for salad and soup rather than the chef's special. And know that you can get back to healthy home eating in a few days.

WHAT HAPPENED:
You twisted your ankle at boot camp, and now you're sidelined for several weeks.

WHAT YOU CAN DO ABOUT IT:
Use this unexpected time to start those home organization projects you've been putting off. Treat it as a mini-vacation, knowing that you'll be back in class in no time.

When we are *consistently flexible,* we trust ourselves to do our best without letting the inevitable hiccups permanently throw us off course. So it's okay to skip a workout in order to see a movie with friends; instead, recognize the importance of reconnecting with those we love. And then make it a victory by returning to the gym the next day.

Life doesn't always go as planned. So, to get where we want to go, we need to do what we can with what we've got at the moment, and consistently keep at it until we get there.

·······················> ╱▔▔▔▔▔▔▔▔▔╲ <·······················
                          │ SOCIAL SHARE │

When we get derailed it can be hard to get back on track.
So think back to a time when you found a way to be
consistently flexible, and then share your snippet with the
community. Or, if you're struggling for even one example,
ask your friends to share their tricks for success. You're
bound to find one that works for you. #wycwyc

BE NON-OBSESSIVELY DETERMINED

• •

LET'S TAKE A LOOK AT ANOTHER FORM OF being flexible: being "non-obsessively determined" in pursuing our goals. Now, this phrase might seem like an oxymoron. And besides, how can we succeed unless we're focused and determined all the time?

There's a difference between being determined and being wholly and utterly *obsessed*. When we're determined we stick to our vision; when we're obsessed, our vision has narrowed so much our goal is all we see—and the rest of life passes us by.

We think life is too short to be dictated by such a myopic perspective.

We urge you not to become so focused on your goals that they get in the way of your *life*. Now, it's a great accomplishment to be committed to, say, going to the gym regularly. But allow yourself to

> We all obsess about what we are doing and accomplishing. What if we let it go and simply made the way we live our lives our accomplishment?
>
> –*Maria Shriver*
>
> #wycwyc

skip a session once in a while when life comes along and offers you another opportunity. Because you know what? It will!

Especially when it comes to fitness, sometimes what we need is rest—so we can refocus. Then we can return more determined, reenergized.

But when healthy living or searching for healthy-living opportunities becomes the only thing we focus on—to the exclusion of friends and family—it can turn into an obsession. And obsessions are never healthy.

When you are non-obsessively determined, and doing WHAT YOU CAN WHEN YOU CAN, it gives you the freedom to *live* as you work toward your goals, with no shortsighted confinement.

Successful WYCWYCers are non-obsessively determined to reach their goals. They do everything in their power to achieve what they set out to achieve, but they also recognize when it's time to raise the white flag—without guilt, without thinking they've failed.

Determination is good. Obsession is not. It's important to know the difference.

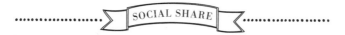

SOCIAL SHARE

Share a recent moment when you walked away from obsession and took a time-out. Show your fellow WYCWYCers it's okay to take a breather once in a while! #wycwyc

BE RESPONSIBLY SELFISH

● ●

BEING SELFISH IS GENERALLY SEEN IN A NEG-ative light, but we'd like to share a different side of selfish. And if there's anything we hope you've learned about wycwyc so far, it's realizing that things aren't always what they seem.

> A red rose is not selfish because it wants to be a red rose. It would be horribly selfish if it wanted all the other flowers in the garden to be both red and roses.
>
> –*Oscar Wilde*
>
> #wycwyc

When you join in the conversation and watch other wycwycers in action, you might notice that those who seem to be the most successful in achieving their goals are the ones who are *responsibly* selfish with their actions.

But what does that mean, being responsibly selfish? It means putting on your oxygen mask before helping others with theirs. Otherwise, to paraphrase one aviation explanation, you might pass out before you can help those less abled—which leaves you all down for the count.

Plus, doing what we need to do to reach our personal goals doesn't just make us healthier, it also makes us happier—which is as much of a win for us as it is for those around us.

While it might seem like a tricky balancing act, it is possible to juggle the needs and wants of others *and* yourself. Consider these scenarios:

WHAT'S THE SITUATION:
Your kids complain that you spend too much time at the gym.

WHAT YOU CAN DO:
Balance your self-care time with your love-care time: promise them an activity of their choosing after you get back.

WHAT'S THE SITUATION:
Your new healthy palate is frustrating your partner.

WHAT YOU CAN DO:
Find a restaurant that caters to both your tastes.

Take that me time to do what makes you feel stronger and more fulfilled. You'll then be in a better position to please and support those around you.

And don't forget that being responsibly selfish doesn't necessarily mean you're putting others last. Making yourself a priority allows you to be the best *you* you can be.

To paraphrase Hillel the Elder: *If I am not for myself, who else will be? But if I am only for myself, what good am I? And if not now, when?*

Get creative. Be responsibly selfish by taking time for yourself AND supporting those around you.

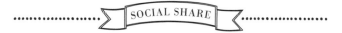

SOCIAL SHARE

Share your responsibly selfish moment with the wycwyc community. How did you meet your needs while balancing them with the interests of friends and family? Spend a few moments encouraging others to do the same. #wycwyc

STOP PARALYSIS BY ANALYSIS

• •

LET'S TAKE SOME Q&A. ANY QUESTIONS FROM the audience?

- ★ "Is doing weights or cardio better for weight loss?"
- ★ "What's the best food plan to follow?"
- ★ "How many times per week should I work out?"
- ★ "Should I exercise before or after work?"

> You can spend minutes, hours, days, weeks or even months overanalyzing a situation; trying to put the pieces together, justifying what could've, would've happened . . . or you can just leave the pieces on the floor and move the f*ck on.
>
> – *Tupac Shakur*
> #wycwyc

So many questions! So much complication! But it's actually pretty simple—there's one answer for all these kinds of wonders and worries: *It doesn't matter.*

("What?")

"It" doesn't matter. What matters is you.

What's the best workout? It doesn't matter.

What matters is that you choose an exercise routine you can commit to. It doesn't matter if studies have shown Workout X is guaranteed to get results more quickly if Workout X is not something you would actually *do*. Between the X you won't end up doing and the Y that you would, clearly the Y is the way to go. And if not Y, then Z. (Be consistently flexible!)

What's the most efficient way to organize your healthy food plan? It doesn't matter.

The best approach is doing WHAT YOU CAN WHEN YOU CAN in a way that fits *your* life. Stop overthinking, overplanning, overplotting, and overanalyzing. Remember: be *non-obsessively* determined. WYCWYC is all about forward momentum—and not allowing yourself to get stuck in the details. It's shifting from planning to *doing*: doing WHAT WE CAN WHEN WE CAN, ever striving to reach our goals.

We know about all this overanalysis because we've done plenty of it ourselves. We've often gotten bogged down researching workout benefits and perfect eating plans. And, to be completely honest, this overplanning has always been more about stalling than anything else. And that's a pretty effective tactic: when we find ourselves stuck overanalyzing options, we usually end up choosing nothing at all.

Real change comes when we look up from the trees and see the forest. For example . . .

WHAT'S THE SITUATION:
Though you did the best you could with the menu at The Burger Shack, you have no idea how many calories you consumed.

WHAT YOU CAN DO ABOUT IT:
Estimate and move on—and don't beat yourself up about it, because you're being flexible!

WHAT'S THE SITUATION:
You have time for only cardio or weight training: which to choose?

WHAT YOU CAN DO ABOUT IT:
Wisely spend the time you do have: go with your gut, pick one, and get on with it!

WHAT'S THE SITUATION:
Your pedometer conked out mid-walk. How can you determine how to meet your daily commitment?

WHAT YOU CAN DO ABOUT IT:
Don't stress about it. Those steps still count—you know they do! Keep moving.

Though paralysis by analysis can take many forms, at the core it's really all the same: a barrier between you and success. We must learn to trust ourselves to make a good choice for today—and know we can always change course tomorrow if today's choice doesn't feel right.

We may misstep here or there, but as long as we're moving forward, we're still making progress.

Stop overanalyzing.

Make a choice.

Onward.

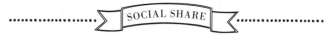
SOCIAL SHARE

Search and scan the #wycwyc hashtag. Notice anyone overanalyzing? Offer them a gentle reminder to stop paralysis by analysis. Remember, we're all in this together! #wycwyc

FAKE IT 'TIL YOU MAKE IT

●●

AHHH, PLAYING MAKE-BELIEVE.

Kids love it. They pretend they're cowboys, or magicians, or dinosaurs.

As adults, we recognize the power of children's pretend play. But we rarely stop and consider its potential for our lives. Playing pretend is just another way to do WHAT YOU CAN WHEN YOU CAN to create the healthy lives we want.

You might have guessed by now that pushing ourselves to live healthier is as much a mind game as it is a body one. A "fake it 'til you make it" strategy can help us win that game: it tricks our brains into believing we're already there! When we harness the powers of visualization, and "see" ourselves living the WYCWYC life we want, we are that much more likely to succeed.

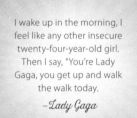

I wake up in the morning, I feel like any other insecure twenty-four-year-old girl. Then I say, "You're Lady Gaga, you get up and walk the walk today.

– *Lady Gaga*

#wycwyc

You may be thinking this sounds implausible. We can remember what it was like to pretend to be a princess or a champion horseback rider, but how exactly do we pretend we're healthy and fit?

It's actually easier than you might think. Well, easy*ish*. Here's how you do it:

CREATE A NARRATIVE

Picture your end goal and imagine you're already there:

- ★ What would you eat for breakfast?

- ★ How would you dress?

- ★ What would you order for lunch at a restaurant?

- ★ How confident would you feel walking down the street?

- ★ How readily would you accept invitations to activities you don't do now?

- ★ What activities would you be doing regularly that you don't do now?

Envision how all areas of your life will look when you're fully living the healthy life you want—and then make a conscious choice to carry yourself as that person, starting *today*.

ENLIST YOUR LOVED ONES

Now it's one thing to visualize yourself; it's another to see ourselves reflected in the eyes of those around us. And, like it or not, other people affirm the way we see ourselves.

So, share your healthy-living goals with those you trust—including the fact that you're utilizing a role-playing strategy in order to visualize your goals coming to fruition. Essentially, this is about asking others to respect the path you've chosen. (We say much more about this in Chapter 16.)

RESPOND AS YOUR FUTURE SELF

Decadent desserts as part of your prix fixe dinner, unpredictable schedules, last-minute deadlines—sometimes it seems the more we try to WYCWYC our lives, the more life intervenes to tempt us away from our best intentions. Trust us: we know how steep our climb can seem when we're just starting out.

But what if we were to respond to all those potential roadblocks as our future selves would? This starts with viewing every situation from a different vantage point: not at the bottom of the mountain, but right at the very top. For example . . .

WHAT'S THE SITUATION:
When faced with a family stop at the ice cream parlor, it can be tough thinking: "I want a waffle cone sundae like the kids are having, but I also want to lose weight . . ." Viewed from that perspective, it's easy to feel overwhelmed by our goals.

WHAT YOU CAN DO ABOUT IT:
But what if you instead thought: "Yeah, I want a waffle cone sundae, but my goals are more important, so I'll get the nonfat frozen yogurt with fresh strawberries."

WHAT'S THE SITUATION:
You're exhausted after a tough day. You'd planned to go to the gym on your way home, but you'd really rather veg out in front of the TV. You tell yourself: "It'll take ages before I'm in shape. What's one less day working out anyway?"

WHAT YOU CAN DO ABOUT IT:
Instead, remind yourself how exercise reenergizes you more than relaxing on the couch does.

Through shifting your thought process—and, as a result, your life-style—your body *will* in time follow your brain. So the *you* you long imagined will start to take shape, until it's fully arrived. You were faking it, but now you're *there.*

Of course, the "future you" will still have to contend with "current you" challenges. When those come up, we urge you to be strong, imagining what you'll feel like further down your healthy-living path. Then, do WHAT YOU CAN WHEN YOU CAN to keep moving forward.

When the going gets tough—the tough start pretending!

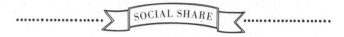
SOCIAL SHARE

Ponder the person you want to become. Today, do one thing your future self would do automatically as a healthy habit, whether it's drinking more water, taking a walk, or getting more sleep. Take a photo and share it with the community! #wycwyc

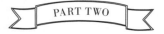

PART TWO

RETHINK AND
TAKE CHARGE

CREATE MARGINS

• •

> "No" is a complete sentence.
>
> – *Anne Lamott*
>
> #wycwyc

WHEN WAS THE LAST TIME you said "no"? Can you remember?

How did it feel? Was it empowering and freeing? Or did you say it with hesitation and guilt?

It's time to talk about boundaries. Drawing them, creating them, and reminding ourselves that saying "no" now and then is a good thing.

Most of us struggle with declining because of the *refusal* inherent in that "no":

★ "No" to extra time after work

★ "No" to partners who want more of our time than we want to give

★ "No" to friends who don't want us to change as we pursue our healthy-living goals

★ "No" to people who simply aren't a priority to us at the moment

Saying "no" can be a valuable tool to help us do What We Can When We Can in prioritizing our healthy-living goals.

•••••••••●•••••••••

When you pause to think about it, it's almost funny how hard it is to say. "No" is such a short word—two letters—yet it can pose such a monumental challenge.

We think the reason it's so hard to respond in the negative is the weight it carries. When we say "no" we are, in fact, telling someone he or she isn't a priority right now. And that can make us uncomfortable—it feels self-centered.

That's okay. This is just another aspect of being responsibly selfish.

When we say "no," we prioritize, we set boundaries. Think of it as words on a page. This page you're reading has space in the margins: free for writing notes if you like, or just to leave open. When you set boundaries around what you'll do for others, you create and reserve space for yourself: adequate time and freedom to DO WHAT YOU CAN with.

Each time you say "yes" to someone else's priorities in place of your own, you cut into the extra space in your life. Once in a while that might be an essential sacrifice, but if it's a habit we'll never achieve our healthy-living goals.

We all have commitments we can't get out of. But once we've harnessed the power of flexibility, we're able to pause and ask ourselves if *this* particular commitment is one we could choose to responsibly decline.

That's the first step: considering if you should say "no." The next part, actually saying it, can be much more difficult. In fact, it's so difficult that we've created a strategy: no matter who is making the request or what the request is—from dreary obligation to fantastic opportunity—we never say "yes" in the moment. This approach gives us the space to consider the impact on our longer-term goals—as well as to figure out if we can flexibly meet everyone's needs. For example . . .

WHAT'S THE REQUEST:
"Can you babysit for us tonight?"

WHAT YOU CAN SAY:
"Let me check my calendar and get back to you."

WHAT'S THE REQUEST:
"Do you want to go to a movie this week?"

WHAT YOU CAN SAY:
"Sounds fun! Let me see if I can get a sitter."

WHAT'S THE REQUEST:
"Could you take over my project while I'm on leave?"

WHAT YOU CAN SAY:
"Let me think about it. I'll want to consult my family first."

Having a default "can't answer yet" response buys us the necessary time to evaluate how the opportunity aligns with our priorities. Because that's what a *yes* is, right? When you agree to something, you articulate that what you've committed to is a priority, for you, right now.

After years of too many *yes*es, we've learned the power of *no*, and it's been unbelievably freeing. It took courage at first, but with each "no" we've established clear boundaries—leaving us space in the margins where we can continue to prioritize our goals.

Now, consider the ripple effect "no" could have on your life and the pursuit of your goals.

When you decide you have the right to set boundaries, to make sure you leave space in the margins for yourself, you're in a better position to do WHAT YOU CAN WHEN YOU CAN to pursue your life choices. And making conscious decisions about your time sets you up for success whether you say "yes" or "no"—because you did so consciously.

We urge you to practice saying "no."

Shout it a few times. Get used to how it sounds. Because it's a valuable tool to help keep you moving forward.

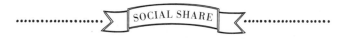

SOCIAL SHARE

Share with the community a time when you created space for yourself by declining a request. #wycwyc

10

STOP TRYING TO BE SOMETHING YOU'RE NOT

• •

IN THE WORLD OF HEALTHY LIVING, IT CAN BE all too easy to get sucked into the next big trend.

Low-carb! CrossFit! Paleo! Zumba! Mud Runs! Detox!

Maybe you've heard stories about a friend of a friend who lost eighty pounds by power walking and eating only cabbage soup. Or another who ran his first marathon after training for a week using some newfangled running program he found online.

We've been there, done that—and failed, plenty of times.

Just because an approach worked for someone else doesn't mean it will work for you. If you hate it, you won't stick with it, and you won't get results. What if you can't stand cabbage? What if you don't like to run? What if avoiding carbs leaves you hungry and stressed? What if training for a 5K with friends sounds like a great way to get fit, but you hate squeezing training sessions into your new work schedule?

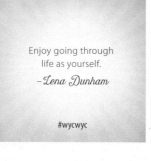

Enjoy going through life as yourself.

–*Lena Dunham*

#wycwyc

Think back to Chapter 7: what's the best workout for you? The one you'll do! Learning to live the WYCWYC way means carving your own path. It means taking into account what others have accomplished—from friends and acquaintances to the self-proclaimed gurus and "experts"—but then making your *own* choices.

Because we have a little secret for you: you're the only expert on you.

Because you are not them. You are unique, and so your healthy-living goals should be tailored to you.

This may sound simplistic, but that's for good reason. There's no need to overcomplicate our lives—they're complicated enough as it is! Just follow your own interests and abilities, be yourself, and good health will follow.

This is not to say you should be passive in your pursuit of healthy-living choices. And, of course, there's something to be said about trying things outside of your comfort zone. Discover what works for you. Put yourself in situations where you can learn about yourself and discover where you excel—and trust your gut along the way. The more you do that, the more your own successful path will take shape.

WYCWYC is about clearly identifying what works for you, your body, and your life, and having the confidence to reach your healthy-living goals on your terms. Self-confidence is like a muscle. In order to be strengthened, you need to sift through the noise, try new things, and give yourself opportunities to discover what works for *you*—not for your cabbage-loving, marathon-running friends.

So stop trying to be something you are not. Just be the expert on you.

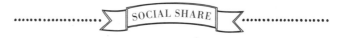

SOCIAL SHARE

Share with the community one new thing you've learned about yourself through doing what you can when you can. #wycwyc

11

TURN YOUR WORDS INSIDE OUT

• •

THE WAY WE THINK DIRECTLY INFLUENCES the way we feel. Consider these examples of how reframing our thoughts might radically shape our lives . . .

> If you cannot make a change, change the way you have been thinking. You might find a new solution.
>
> –*Maya Angelou*
>
> #wycwyc

WHAT WE MAY THINK NOW:
OMG, eating healthy means I can't have all those yummy things I really love.

WHAT WE CAN THINK INSTEAD:
Look at all this healthy food I've never tried before—I might discover a new fave!

WHAT WE MAY THINK NOW:
I don't want to get up early to work out tomorrow.

WHAT WE CAN THINK INSTEAD:
Tomorrow morning I'm making time for myself to de-stress!

It may seem like mere semantics or insignificant details, but these small tweaks in phrasing—even when they're only expressed internally—can greatly affect our overall mindset.

We've talked a lot about the idea of healthy habits. Well, guess what? Cultivating the practice of turning our negative words and thoughts inside out just might be the healthiest habit of all—and possibly the hardest one, too. Why is that?

It's become popular to do the literal or figurative eye roll to all things "healthy," and to commiserate over how hard healthy living is. But the trouble is, the more we think or say something—like "ugh, healthy"—the more likely it is we'll create just that reality.

But it doesn't have to be that way. While self-fulfilling prophecies can generally be negative, we can harness them to propel us closer to achieving healthy-living goal success. Pay attention to both your internal monologue and the words you choose to speak out loud, and notice how they directly affect your efforts:

* "Eating healthier isn't forced deprivation; it's a way to honor my body."

* "Eating a cookie doesn't mean I'm weak; it just means I wanted a cookie."

* "Working out isn't a punishment; it's a way to celebrate my healthy life!"

The more we reframe these acts of healthy living into positive contexts, the more we will start to believe the beneficial messages we're telling ourselves. In fact, this is just another way to fake it 'til we make it!

Our words can affect how we feel, and sometimes doing WHAT WE CAN WHEN WE CAN simply means to choose those words deliberately and with passion, even—no, *especially* on those days when we don't feel like it. When we change the way we think about healthy living, we live with more excitement, motivation, and anticipation.

Positivity, people. It's powerful!

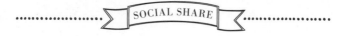

SOCIAL SHARE

Think of something you usually spin negatively, like the "I don't want to get up early to work out" line above. Now, consciously rephrase this thought to turn it into a positive. Then share it with the community! #wycwyc

STOP MUSTURBATING

• •

WE KNEW THIS ONE WOULD CATCH YOUR EYE.

MUSTurbating is something we all do, even though if asked, we'd probably deny it. Coined by Albert Ellis, "MUSTurbating" is an unconscious word habit that can have negative effects on our lives.

Consider these words:

★ Must ★ Should ★ Ought

Now, quickly, make up a separate sentence for each word.

Any of the following sound familiar?

> There are three musts that hold us back: I must do well. You must treat me well. And the world must be easy.
> – *Albert Ellis*,
> American psychologist and founder of Rational Emotive Behavior Therapy
>
> #wycwyc

★ "I must make sure the house is spotless and all chores are done before I take time for myself."

★ "I should lose weight."

★ "I ought to go to the gym every day or I'm never going to reach my fitness goals."

Can you guess how frequently you say these words? And when was the last time you used them without feeling some guilt or anxiety?

A lot of MUSTurbation derives from feeling we need to be perfect. Our strong desires and goals can readily morph into the absolutes of *must* and *should*. These are heavy demands—especially when perfect is *never going to happen*.

And don't think we haven't been there ourselves. Not only have we MUSTurbated into puddles of guilt; we've also dragged along its BFF: shame. Shame likes to tell us we're not good enough—we're broken, defective, lazy, embarrassing to ourselves and our families.

We've decided that guilt and shame are no longer welcome houseguests. We've sent them packing! Now, instead, we go with the flow and do WHAT WE CAN WHEN WE CAN to reach our goals. We WYCWYCers make the choice to turn "must" into "want to," "could," "might," and "I'll consider."

This shift in framework removes self-judgment and returns control back to us, which frees us to progress. Our "musts," "shoulds," and "oughts" have become

* "I wish I had more time to make sure the house is spotless and all laundry and dishes are done."

* "I'm setting a goal to lose a few pounds."

* "I'd love to go to the gym every day but sometimes life gets in the way."

And then, if it doesn't happen, we move on.

That's all. No penalty.

Combating MUSTurbation calls for the same tactics used when we "turn our words inside out": fine-tuning our awareness of this perfectionist mindset. We encourage you to start to notice these pesky little words in both yourself and others.

If you find that you frequently say "must," "should," or "ought," make it a game to catch yourself when you do. Then recast those perfectionistic thoughts in a positive light—and reward yourself for doing so.

We place a lot of unnecessary pressure on ourselves. We wycwyc-ers believe it's time to stop. Let's give up the "musts," "shoulds," and "oughts" altogether.

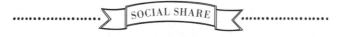
SOCIAL SHARE

Make today's social exercise about the MUSTurbation apparent in others. Read through any social media platform and really notice the words people use. Do any "shoulds" or "musts" catch your eye? Practice being someone else's cheerleader and gently help her reframe her thoughts in positive terms instead. #wycwyc

13

DON'T SETTLE; SEIZE!

ONE OF THE MOST IMPORTANT ASPECTS OF WYCWYC is an emphasis on not settling. Just the opposite: doing WHAT YOU CAN WHEN YOU CAN is about seizing every opportunity to succeed!

WYCWYC is about shifting how you view your entire world and *seizing* everything you can to move forward toward success. It's about being honest with yourself and having the confidence to pursue WHAT YOU CAN in all ways—even when it's scary, or overwhelming, or risky, or out of your everyday pattern.

> There is no passion to be found playing small—in settling for a life that is less than the one you are capable of living.
>
> – *Nelson Mandela*
>
> #wycwyc

Those who do WHAT THEY CAN WHEN THEY CAN harness all opportunities, no matter how small or seemingly insignificant.

We like to think of seizing the moment as reaching up and yanking an apple (healthy!) from a tree. Now, if we'd waited, the apple would fall on its own eventually, but who has time for that? Seize the apple!

Need some examples of how you can seize your WYCWYC day?

wycwyc is healthy living,
carpe diem – style!

·············●●·············

WHAT'S THE SITUATION:
You're stuck at the mechanic's waiting for an oil change.

WHAT YOU CAN DO ABOUT IT:
Come on, don't sit in the waiting room reading outdated magazines. Take a walk! Better yet, go for a jog!

WHAT'S THE SITUATION:
Have tons of laundry to haul upstairs?

WHAT YOU CAN DO ABOUT IT:
Skip the basket and take multiple trips! Or go all out: set a timer and race yourself up the stairs. Got kids? Race them up the stairs!

WHAT'S THE SITUATION:
Forgot to defrost something for dinner?

WHAT YOU CAN DO ABOUT IT:
Enlist the family in a challenge: raid the pantry and come up with a crazy-fun dinner.

Making an effort to seize every opportunity you can could look different every day. And that's part of the fun! wycwycers are determined to find and snag every little chance to edge them toward their goals.

Besides, how often has settling for the bare minimum helped anyone achieve success?

Don't settle for a life you don't want. Seize all opportunities and make the life you do want.

Carpe wycwyc!

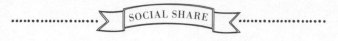

SOCIAL SHARE

Snap a photo of a WYCWYC moment you seized today and share it with the community. Then, tag a few friends and challenge them to document their seized WYCWYC moments, too. #wycwyc

14

QUIT AND MOVE ON

• •

THINK BACK TO CHAPTER 2: WHAT DID WE SAY is one of the most important aspects of WYCWYC living? Persistence.

So, let's say you want to get more fit, and you decide running is the best exercise for you: hey, it's free, right? And you can easily fit it in around your busy schedule. Great; you start your new WYCWYC practice.

Now let's imagine that, several weeks in, running doesn't seem to be working out so well after all: your knees and feet hurt a lot, and you've come to dread the sight of your running shoes.

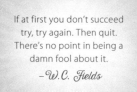

If at first you don't succeed try, try again. Then quit. There's no point in being a damn fool about it.

–W.C. Fields

#wycwyc

But then again, we urge you to be persistent in your goal to be healthy. What *should* you do? Force yourself to continue something you don't like, um, hate? No. What's left: quit?

Quit? How would that be being persistent? And besides, we live in a quitters-never-win-and-winners-never-quit society. And you don't want to be a loser, um, quitter.

But what if quitting running is exactly what you need? What if quitting would actually serve you better than persevering?

Knowing when to quit and move on is a skill we wycwycers work to master. The key is remembering that quitting is the right choice if it saves us time and anguish and opens up space for new and better healthy experiences.

Maybe you gave a workout routine a try and it didn't suit you. Or maybe it *did* suit you—for a while—and now it doesn't. That's okay—nothing lasts forever.

What's important is learning to trust ourselves to know when something isn't working—and then to doing WHAT WE CAN about it. For example . . .

WHAT'S THE SITUATION:
You want to exercise but you really hate running.

WHAT YOU CAN DO ABOUT IT:
Sign up for step class at the gym instead. Maybe exercising in a group is more your style.

WHAT'S THE SITUATION:
You want to start moving more, but it's really hard—you haven't exercised in years, and you get tired really quickly.

WHAT YOU CAN DO ABOUT IT:
Do what you can! Start small by walking and increase your distance slowly.

WHAT'S THE SITUATION:
You want to work out, but you find exercise really boring.

WHAT YOU CAN DO ABOUT IT:
Sign up for a pole-dancing class. (Now that is *not* boring!)

Living the WYCWYC way means having the confidence and strength to shed habits and goals if they no longer serve you. And doing that is also an example of being flexibly consistent. If you refuse to "quit" running but end up running less and less, you're no longer pursuing your goals. But if you quit and *move on* to try a different exercise, you're still consistently, persistently pursuing a healthy lifestyle.

> The first rule of holes: When you're in one, stop digging.
>
> – *Molly Ivins*
>
> #wycwyc

Plus, wise quitting really is the epitome of WYCWYC self-care. It's trusting yourself enough to know when you're making the right choice.

Let's review that because it's important.

It's about trust. Trust in yourself.

Trust that you are the expert of what you need— and that includes what you don't need.

> SOCIAL SHARE

Think about a healthy goal you set a while back that no longer serves you. How might you "quit" an aspect of this goal to reenergize you in its pursuit? Share with the community how you've quit and then revamped. #wycwyc

15

DON'T EXPECT–ASK!

● ●

IT'S TIME TO BE HONEST WITH YOURSELF.

Brutally honest. Candid. Truthful. Even blunt.

Successful wycwycers have the strength to acknowledge, to ourselves and to others:

"I need help managing and juggling life's responsibilities."

But note that asking for help doesn't mean we're weak; just the opposite. It means we're both strong enough and self-aware enough to seek the support we need to succeed.

The trick is, it's tricky! This sort of thing is not as simple as ABC. That's why we're here to walk you through the process of asking for help.

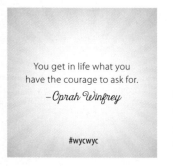

You get in life what you have the courage to ask for.
– *Oprah Winfrey*

#wycwyc

1: NO ONE CAN READ YOUR MIND.

We've all experienced frustration, perhaps even anger, because a loved one was not able to meet our needs by reading our minds. For example:

* "My friend should have known I'd miss my yoga class if she didn't pick up my daughter."

* "My partner should have seen how exhausted I was and helped me make dinner."

* "I've told my family I'm trying to eat healthier. They should have included other food at the potluck."

Do you see a pattern with the above examples? Do you spot that pesky MUSTurbating word we want to avoid?

And should they really be able to read our minds? No. Which leads us to the next item.

2: ASKING FOR HELP CAN BE HARD.

Part of living a WYCWYC lifestyle is acknowledging that the world will not fall apart if we don't manage every single detail ourselves—and trusting that others in our lives are capable of doing some things for us. This calls for doing something a lot of us find hard: delegating.

Terrifying to so many of us, delegating is a necessary WYCWYC skill if you want to create space in your life for self-care.

In addition:

3: WE NEED TO COMMUNICATE OUR NEEDS.

To effectively ask others for help, we'll want to clearly communicate our needs. And the most important piece of learning to do that is first *defining* exactly what it is we need.

Compare the following requests with the mind-reading examples we shared earlier:

- ★ "Would you pick up my daughter so I can be on time for yoga?"

- ★ "I'm beat. Can you handle dinner tonight?"

- ★ "Can you bring your famous healthy salad to the potluck? I'm trying to eat healthier."

Do you see how these questions not only ask for help but also clearly state *how* others can help? And for those of us squeamish about delegating, consider something else: there's more to delegating than just relinquishing control.

Defining for others precisely how they can help you makes your life a bit easier by creating those margins we've talked about—which gives you the time and space to seize more WYCWYC opportunities. So learn to delegate. Learn to ask. You can't do everything—and, really, even if you could, why would you?

Asking for help doesn't have to be just task-oriented. Another key to WYCWYC success is encouragement, and lots of it. Sometimes we need a cheerleader to remind us we've got this! So ideally we'll learn to ask for emotional support when we need more than we're getting. For example:

"I don't know if I can stay strong tomorrow in the face of Betty's birthday cake. Remind me I really don't want it; remind me it's not worth it."

That's a simpler one. But sometimes we need to articulate more specifically the phrasing we'll respond to. For example, consider this exchange:

"I'm exhausted. I'm not sure I can finish the boot camp series. Tell me I can do this."
"You can do this."
"Uh, can you try louder?"

"You can do this!"
"More!"
"You can do this!! Only four more boot camp sessions!"

Now, we know asking for help might seem too hard on those days when you're feeling depleted, but it does get easier. And when you ask for support as with the boot camp above, it's more than worth it.

And, it just so happens that some of your requests will be welcome. Haven't you wanted to help a family member with an ailing parent or a newborn, but not known how? Well, we bet there's people in your life who have felt the same way about you. Enlist them to play a role in your healthy-living narrative, and build your supporting cast!

But wait, there's one last pitfall we need to mention:

4: IT WON'T ALWAYS WORK.

We wish it would—but if we've learned anything from wycwycing, it's that we control only ourselves. Everyone else is on their own journeys. But that doesn't mean we don't ask.

Ask!

You may or may not receive, but the rewards are great when you do.

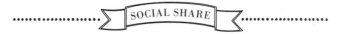

Take a risk. Stop and ask online wycwyc friends for help or share how you asked for help offline. Be the example and show others that asking for help is a sign of strength, not weakness. #wycwyc

CHOOSE FRIENDS WISELY

● ●

WE ARE THE SUM OF THOSE WHO SURROUND us. Each person we choose to spend time with influences us—who we are, and who we become.

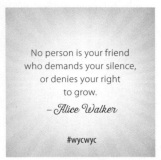

No person is your friend who demands your silence, or denies your right to grow.

– *Alice Walker*

#wycwyc

Think about the people you spend time with. What fantastic traits do they have that you'd like to adopt? What traits—and be honest—of theirs potentially have a negative effect on your goals?

WYCWYC is all about pursuing healthy paths and snagging what healthy-living opportunities we find along the way. Now, do the people you surround yourself with promote that effort, or do they hinder it? Are they your cheerleaders, or are they naysayers? Do they support you, or do they discourage you?

We often don't consider so closely the company we keep, especially in how those around us affect the pursuit of our goals. But once we're in the process of carving our healthy-living path, it would be wise to pay closer attention to the impacts of our social interactions.

Notice who encourages. Notice who discourages. Who offers a helping hand? Who always tries to outdo? For example, consider the following:

* "You don't need to go to the gym today. Let's go out to eat instead."
* "Let's treat ourselves to ice cream. We deserve it. It's been a long week."

Now we're not saying comments like these are intentionally unsupportive. It's just that some people's priorities simply don't match ours. That's okay! We don't have to break off these relationships—we can still enjoy them for other attributes. What we *can* do is surround ourselves with a supportive inner circle.

Once we identify who in our network is receptive to our healthy-living efforts, and who is resistant, we're better able to choose who will be in that circle—as well as to lessen, as much as possible, the interactions we share with those we can't walk away from.

We WYCWYCers surround ourselves with teams of people who really want us to succeed—some of whom we've never even met! Sometimes doing WHAT YOU CAN WHEN YOU CAN means taking the step to reach out online—via social media—to find the support you need to succeed in your healthy-living efforts.

Remember, who you surround yourself with is a *choice*. Choose wisely.

.... ⟩ SOCIAL SHARE ⟨ ....

Reach out to a new friend today, someone you may not know offline but have spied on social media. Offer support. Ask for encouragement. Start conversations. Friendship is all about baby steps. Tag with the hashtag so you inspire others to forge new friendships as well. #wycwyc

TRY NEW THINGS
CONSISTENTLY

• •

CONSIDER YOUR ANSWERS TO THE FOLLOWING questions:

> Courage and willingness to just go for it, whether it is a conversation or a spontaneous trip or trying new things that are scary—it is a really attractive quality.
>
> – *Alanis Morissette*
>
> #wycwyc

* Who are you?

* What do you like?

* What do you dislike?

* What are you good at?

* What are you absolutely, unequivocally terrible at?

Do you have all your answers?

Great—now forget all of it!

Before we can truly rock the WYCWYC life, we need to stop, step back, and loosen our attachment to our self-definitions.

For example, think about some of the things you say about yourself:

- "I'm not good at volleyball. I was humiliated in high school gym class because I couldn't serve over the net."

- "The company softball team looks really fun, but I'm not athletic that way."

- "I'd love to try out these healthy recipes and host a dinner party for all my coworkers, but I'm not a great cook."

Though our sense of who we are, what we like, and how we act has been defined in part by our life experiences, that doesn't mean we need to stick with those definitions.

Nor do we have to let others define us. For example, consider the following:

- "I didn't ask if you wanted to participate in our 5K event because I know you're not a runner."

- "I organized a group outing to the farmers' market but I know that's not your thing."

- "I assumed you wouldn't like my potluck dinner idea because you always go out to eat."

The trouble is, it's all too easy to internalize these kinds of messages. The end result can be a self-definition that tremendously limits our persistence in trying new things in the pursuit of our goals.

Doing WHAT YOU CAN WHEN YOU CAN sometimes calls for taking a leap of faith when your self-definition is holding you back. For example, let's revisit the earlier scenarios:

- "Though I usually walk when I do a 5K, I think this weekend I might try to jog a bit as well."

- "Even though I grew up hating vegetables, I'm committed to trying one new veg-based recipe a week."

★ "I've always been an introvert by nature, but today I'll try reaching-ing out to people in the WYCWYC community."

Remember when we told you to say "no!" and live with your margins? Now you're ready to start saying "YES!"

Say "yes" to new opportunities.

Say "yes" to new experiences.

Say "yes" to things that may surprise those around you.

Say "yes" to things that will stretch your self-definition.

To get the ball rolling, it might be helpful to choose a day or week or even a month when you're open to trying almost everything that comes your way.

For example, imagine accepting the following invitations . . .

WHAT'S THE OFFER:

"Want to try this new recipe with me?"

WHAT YOU CAN REPLY:

"Absolutely!"

WHAT'S THE OFFER:

"I want to challenge myself to run one of those obstacle races."

WHAT YOU CAN REPLY:

"You know what? That's a great idea. Count me in too."

WHAT'S THE OFFER:

"Josh is starting a running group. Would you like to join us now and then?"

WHAT YOU CAN REPLY:

"Sure! I'd love to."

We like to say, "I'm in!"

The more frequently you encounter new experiences, the more you'll be able to snag healthy-living moments. And when you're really living the WYCWYC life, you'll notice all sorts of opportunities around you—but first you have to be open to experiencing them.

You'll never know what new things you might love until you *try*.

We're in. Are you? Join us!

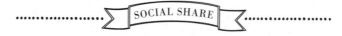

SOCIAL SHARE

It's time to push yourself out of your comfort zone. Try something for the first time today, then announce it to the community. You may inspire someone to try something new as well. #wycwyc

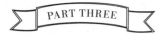
PART THREE

DAILY
CONSIDERATIONS

18

MAXIMIZE
YOUR EFFORT

● ●

TO USE A WELL-WORN PHRASE, IT'S TIME TO kill two birds with one stone.

We tend to plow through life carrying laundry lists of things we *need* to do. Things we *need* to accomplish.

We also have lists upon lists of things we *want* to do. Experiences we *want* to have.

What if we could combine these needs with the wants? It might look something like this:

> Most people are so busy knocking themselves out trying to do everything they think they should do, they never get around to what they want to do.
>
> – *Kathleen Winsor*,
> author of *Forever Amber*
>
> #wycwyc

★ "I need to restock the fridge, but I really want to spend time with my partner. Hmm: we could meet up at the farmers' market!"

★ "I know the laundry's piling up, but I'd rather spend time with the kids. I know, we'll have a contest to see who can sort the clothes fastest!"

★ "I really want to go for a run, but I haven't seen my friends in weeks. I wonder if Susy would be up for a running date on that new trail."

Can you see how these scenarios could help you maximize your efforts? With just a little creativity, the drudgery of to-do lists can turn into fun!

Maximizing our efforts is all about marrying our wants with our needs.

Now some want-and-need pairings will come naturally; others won't be so obvious. It takes an open-minded, creative approach to see how easily things like dates and dry cleaning or friends and farmers' markets can go together.

Of course, not all things lend themselves to multitasking; sometimes monotasking is the way to go. You're the expert on you, and you'll come to know the difference.

But the times when we can double up can be exhilarating! We accomplish more while making the most of our time, maximizing our efforts.

It's a win-win.

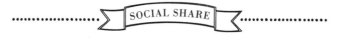

Take a photo of yourself rocking the fun multitask. Then share it with the community! #wycwyc

19

SWAP PASSIVE FOR ACTIVE

• •

WE DON'T KNOW ABOUT YOURS, BUT OUR childhoods were action-packed. Running outside. Jumping up the stairs. Racing to the car. Not to mention playing sports and dancing to the radio.

We'd go nonstop and think nothing of it.

> Don't give up. Keep going. There is always a chance that you stumble onto something terrific. I have never heard of anyone stumbling over anything while . . . sitting down.
>
> – *Ann Landers*
>
> #wycwyc

Now that we're adults, however, everything we do seems to be passive by default. Sitting at a desk. Kicking back in front of the TV. Watching sports rather than playing them. And any surfing we do is strictly on the Web.

Did you learn in school that an object at rest stays at rest? Well, now *we're* those objects.

Adopting a WYCWYC mindset calls for no longer defaulting to inactivity. The more we do WHAT WE CAN, the more we learn to swap out those passive activities for more active ones. It's all part of consciously *moving* through our lives. The good news is that movement begets movement!

The more we WYCWYC our world and maintain activity, the more our bodies crave this movement.

Swapping passive for active can be as simple as

- ★ Investing in a standing desk for your home office

- ★ Swapping your book club meetings on the couch for a walking discussion

- ★ Snagging some steps walking around the room while you talk on that long conference call

- ★ Doing wall sits while brushing your teeth

- ★ Holding a plank position for few moments when reading

- ★ Trying a *run*ch date—chat over a run and then go for smoothies

- ★ Taking a walk to de-stress instead of vegging in front of the TV

- ★ Taking your date roller skating, bowling, or rock climbing

- ★ Taking fitness breaks, not coffee breaks

- ★ Standing instead of sitting on the subway, or, better yet, getting off a stop or two early

When you begin making choices like these on a daily basis, swapping passive for active becomes a healthy habit. And, in true WYCWYC form, once you start to view your world through this lens, the more opportunities will present themselves.

We just thought of one . . .

How about taking a walk and thinking about this chapter?

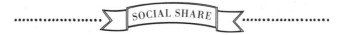

SOCIAL SHARE

Share through a photo or video a creative way you've transformed something passive into something active. Tag it with #wycwyc #swap so we can find and share your fun ideas. #wycwyc

EMBRACE DECONVENIENCE

• •

OUR LIVES HAVE BECOME TOO DARN CONVENIENT.
Smart phones. Remote controls. Escalators. Grocery delivery.

It all rocks—until we pause and recognize how all this convenience adds up to an increasingly sedentary life. How many extra steps do we miss out on each day by virtue of our modern lives?

Okay, we may not be ready to entirely surrender all our modern conveniences. We don't all want to grow our own food or hand wash our clothes. But that doesn't mean our lives have to be convenient just for convenience's sake.

> An escalator can never break: it can only become stairs. You should never see an ESCALATOR TEMPORARILY OUT OF ORDER sign, just ESCALATOR TEMPORARILY STAIRS. SORRY FOR THE CONVENIENCE.
>
> – *Mitch Hedberg*
>
> #wycwyc

There doesn't always have to be an easy way, especially when that easy way steals simple opportunities from us to be more active!

Consider setting up your home to create an environment that allows you to move in ways you wouldn't otherwise. We know it may

When we look for fun ways to deconvenience instead of always seeking shortcuts, we begin to see the positive advantages of our extra effort.

••••••••••●●•••••••••

sound counterintuitive, but that's only because it's part of our society's mindset to look for shortcuts.

* Why walk when we could ride?

* Why carry when we could push?

* Why get out of the car when we could just drive through?

Why indeed? It's a fun challenge to find ways that *de*conveniencing our surroundings can further reinforce the WYCWYC behaviors we seek. And then tally them up. For example . . .

WHAT WE DO NOW:
Carry a basket of dirty clothes to the laundry room.

WHAT WE COULD DO INSTEAD:
Carry individual piles of clothes! How many more steps would you take if you skipped the laundry basket?

WHAT WE DO NOW:
Change the TV channel with the remote control.

WHAT WE COULD DO INSTEAD:
Place the remote control across the room when watching television. How much more would you move if the TV remote was across the room?

WHAT WE DO NOW:
Use the closest bathroom.

WHAT WE COULD DO INSTEAD:
Use the bathroom that's farthest away. How much would your step count increase if you pretended the closest restroom didn't exist? Bonus points if the farther one is on a different floor!

Doing WHAT YOU CAN to deconvenience requires some personal creativity, and will vary depending on your environment, be it an apartment or a ranch-style home. Either way, keep in mind that deconvenience isn't about making things more *difficult*. It's simply about seeing the inherent value of our efforts and recognizing that everything counts toward our fulfilling our goals—even taking just one extra flight of stairs a day.

We challenge you to join us in the fight against modern convenience just for convenience's sake. Every time you do something, every time you make a move, challenge yourself with this question: "How might I make this a bit less convenient and a lot more rewarding?"

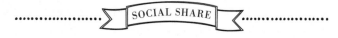

SOCIAL SHARE

Snap a photo of your best or most outrageous deconvenient idea and share it with the community. #wycwyc

ACTIVATE YOUR WAIT TIMES

CONSIDER HOW MUCH TIME WE SPEND WAITING:

* For the coffee to brew

* For the meeting to begin

* For the email reply

* For our turn to see the doctor

* For the elevator to open

* For customer service to answer

* For the class to let out

* For the light to turn green

* For the checkout line to move

* For the server to take our order

* For the movie to start

> We must use time wisely and forever realize that the time is always ripe to do right.
>
> – *Nelson Mandela*
>
> #wycwyc

These wait times could seem frustrating—until you start to view them as opportunities in disguise. We WYCWYCers love to make otherwise mundane moments work in our favor, and there's nothing more mundane than waiting.

Let's reclaim that waiting time! The WYCWYC mindset encourages us to take advantage of all those previously "wasted" moments to our benefit. Instead of complaining we don't have time for fitness, or self-care, or connecting with friends, how about reinventing the portions of our days spent waiting for something? For example . . .

WHAT WE DO NOW:
Idly peruse old magazines while waiting at the mechanic.

WHAT WE COULD DO INSTEAD:
Call an old friend and take a stroll while chatting.

WHAT WE DO NOW:
Stand around waiting for the microwave to beep/the water to boil/the toast to pop.

WHAT WE COULD DO INSTEAD:
See how many counter push-ups we can complete.

WHAT WE DO NOW:
Think of repetitive tasks like weeding or cleaning as drudgery.

WHAT WE COULD DO INSTEAD:
Rethink these as great opportunities for mindful meditation.

Now, you might think five extra minutes spent working toward your healthy-living goals isn't a big deal. Really? Spread out over three or four times a day, seven days a week, those extra minutes add up pretty quickly. This won't prepare you to run a marathon, but the reinforced mindset definitely prepares you for whatever you pursue: diet and exercise, self-care—you name it. And don't forget: any action you take toward lessening your stress level and increasing your productivity is good for your health and happiness.

Time is too precious to waste. What are you *waiting* for?

⟩ SOCIAL SHARE ⟨

Snag a quick video of yourself seizing some wait time. Feeling shy? Film only your feet! #wycwyc

22

PENCIL IT IN!

• •

NOW, WE WANT TO TAKE A MOMENT TO CLAR-
ify a few things. Clearly the wycwyc mindset is wholly and utterly
about *going with the flow*. We want you to seize every opportunity
that presents itself; we urge you to rethink ways to fit in those baby
steps; and we remind you that sometimes quitting something
that isn't working is the best way to
move forward.

> The key is not to prioritize
> what's on your schedule,
> but to schedule
> your priorities.
>
> *– Stephen Covey*
>
> #wycwyc

Though we may let go of the idea that
we're striving for perfection, that doesn't
mean we have no idea what our routine would actually look like in a perfect
world. And even though we know few
weeks will transpire without a hitch, we
still plan our time as though they will. We
just plan in pencil!

Any success expert will tell you no one achieved a great goal without planning and plotting how to complete it. For us it's no different:
having a guideline of what we want to accomplish in each day or

If we have no sense of where we want to end up, it's certain we won't get there.

•••••••••●●●••••••••

each week is essential to achieving our goals. We just pursue those daily or weekly goals WYCWYC-style!

That means regularly asking yourself whether you can realistically squeeze any you time moments into your day or week. However you like to schedule your time—in a datebook, online, or on the back of your morning muffin napkin—make it a habit to include a WYCWYC entry on your to-do list. Successful WYCWYC scheduling is fluid scheduling because we know life has a habit of derailing our best-laid plans. By remaining fluid, *penciling* things in, we still keep track of our goals and know where we're headed, even if our path getting there is somewhat crooked.

Consider the following . . .

WHAT WE DO NOW:
Schedule a run on Monday, Wednesday, and Friday.

WHAT WE COULD DO INSTEAD:
Pencil in three runs, probably Monday, Wednesday, and Friday, but if not, have Saturday morning open, too—and a bit of time Sunday afternoon.

Success comes not from strict perfectionism and tightly adhering to your calendar, but from doing WHAT YOU CAN WHEN YOU CAN, and knowing why you're doing it.

And some days and weeks we'll finish as we hoped we would, with a resounding *Check, check, check! Did it all!*

Other days and weeks won't turn out just as we'd planned, and that's okay too.

It's up to you how strict you want to be about your healthy goal timeline. Some may prefer to schedule WYCWYC moments more as business appointments—and then fiercely protect those time slots. Others may prefer to plot their time more loosely, expecting the likely shifts and changes to the master plan. Regardless of your approach, don't let your inner pesky perfectionist act up if things don't go quite as you'd hoped.

Keep that eraser handy!

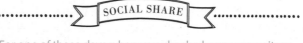

SOCIAL SHARE

For one of those days when you checked your WYCWYC item off your list: First, pat yourself on the back! Then, share your success with the community. You'll likely inspire someone else to seize her moment as well! #wycwyc

23

WALK THIS WAY

• •

WALKING IS SLOW. IT JUST IS.

Even the swiftest walker among us is not as fast as the slowest vehicle.

But you know what?

We wycwyers don't care. You could even say we like it that way! Why?

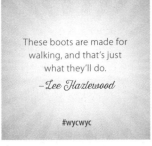

These boots are made for walking, and that's just what they'll do.

–Lee Hazlewood

#wycwyc

* Walking helps us slow down, giving us time to think, savor life, and enjoy the little things.

* Walking is an easy way to get us moving. It doesn't require any special equipment or training.

* Walking is convenient. We can do it rain or shine, alone or in a group.

* Walking is free. And we can save money by walking instead of driving or taking the bus or subway.

*Sometimes getting in the car
is more habit than necessity.
What if your habit
were walking instead?*

........●●●........

Come to think of it, why aren't we walking as much as possible?

A big facet of WHAT YOU CAN WHEN YOU CAN is seizing the opportunity to move and walk whenever possible, speed be damned. *Any* forward movement is a win! We believe so much in the power of our feet we'd like to shout Nancy Sinatra loud and clear: your boots were made for walkin'!

Those of us who don't live in urban areas are prone to forget that walking can actually be a mode of transportation. Do you ever take the opportunity to walk somewhere when you'd normally drive?

Take a step back (pun intended!) and think about what may be walkable in your neighborhood. Let's say there's a grocery store or farmers' market about a mile from home. What if you were to get a pushcart or wagon and maximize your effort: combine your Sunday shopping trip with a nice walk?

If you have kids, how far away is their school? Have you considered walking with them one morning a week, or meeting them halfway on their walk home?

In our increasingly convenient society, we're practically likely to hop in the car and ride to the end of the driveway just to get the mail. It's a real shame, too, because not only does walking get you moving, but it can also relax and reenergize you.

We're not exaggerating to tell you that adding walking to our regular repertoire was a real game changer for us. We used to drive, drive, drive. But then we added a pause to our default mode of transportation. Each time we reached for the car keys, we stopped and challenged ourselves with the question "Could this trip be walked?"

Or, at the very least, walked partially?

We're also fans of driving farther than we have to, parking, and walking back to where we need to be. Why fight for that spot right by the grocery store doors when you can leisurely park at the far end of the lot and stroll your way to the market?

All this extra walking opened up an entirely new WYCWYC world for us, and our step counts prove it! We invite you to join us and encourage you to make the most of it. Wave to people you pass, and invite others to walk this way with you. You never know: the more we all choose to walk as a mode of transportation, the more we, as a movement, may begin to shift how our culture views walking. We WYCWYCers can be trailblazers.

We're walking pioneers! Walk!

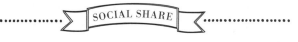

Take a walk. Snap a photo of something you never noticed before and share it with the community. WYCWYC isn't just about fitness. It's also about stopping and smelling the roses—and maybe even making new friends along the way. #wycwyc

BE PREPARED!

● ●

EVERY GIRL SCOUT KNOWS PREPAREDNESS IS the key to success.

In a way, living a wycwyc life prepares you to handle pretty much any obstacle on your healthy-living journey. We're ready to negotiate anything life throws at us, and make those unexpected life events work *with* rather than against our own needs and goals. But there's more to being prepared than just being mentally ready.

Consider: How many times have you not been able to snag a wycwyc opportunity when it presented itself? Have you thought things like the following?

> I believe luck is preparation meeting opportunity. If you hadn't been prepared when the opportunity came along, you wouldn't have been lucky.
>
> *—Oprah Winfrey*
>
> #wycwyc

★ "I would have loved to walk with her at lunch, but I only have my heels at the office."

★ "My stomach was growling, and the only option I had was the vending machine."

* "I was stuck in traffic on the way home—I guess we're having pizza for dinner."

Luckily, these scenarios can often be easily avoided by taking just a few preparatory steps. For example:

* Keep a change of clothes, toiletries, and an old pair of sneakers in your trunk.

* Stash in your desk an emergency kit of healthy nonperishable snacks.

* Stock your pantry with healthy go-to items for pulling together last-minute meals.

* Cook larger dinners and freeze the leftovers for easy lunches.

* On the weekends stock the fridge with grabbable items that will last you all week.

* If you often make last-minute trips, keep a travel bag stocked with resistance bands, a jump rope, and a workout DVD.

* Familiarize yourself with a few different walking paths around your office so you'll know which route to take depending on how much time you have free.

Healthy living isn't always easy, but when we're thinking ahead and preparing for it, the opportunities multiply. In a very tangible way, being prepared allows us to discover even more WYCWYC moments than we would otherwise.

But how do you prepare for the unexpected? Good question! Remember the whole notion of you being the expert on you? It applies here, too. Think about the activities that might call to you, and consider what preparation would allow you to take advantage of unexpected openings in your schedule. You may find all you need is a pair of sneakers and a bottle of water in your trunk. Or maybe hairbands and a dry shirt to change into afterward.

No matter what being prepared means for us individually, it's an important concept to master as we WYCWYC our way to success.

But, just as important as it is to have the *things* we need to reach our goals—sneakers, healthy snacks—we also need to be prepared to use them, and that requires a certain level of self-honesty.

Ask yourself this question:

"Do I let lack of preparation stop me from exercising or eating healthfully?"

Now, this sentence is a mouthful, so take it slowly: we need to be ready to dodge the temptation to skip WYCWYC opportunities. Are you prepared to say "yes" when a coworker invites you to walk around the block? Okay, you have your sneakers, but do you have your WYCWYC attitude too?

This isn't to say that to decline sometimes means you're not walking the WYCWYC talk. We just urge you to be clear on *why* you're saying "no," and that you're not using lack of preparation as an excuse for declining.

Of course, you can't and won't always say yes to every chance that comes your way. However, if you are truly doing WHAT YOU CAN WHEN YOU CAN, you don't need excuses. If you can't, then don't; it's as easy as that.

There's one more angle we want to share. Being prepared is not just about helping ourselves.

Being part of the #wycwyc community means being prepared to help others on their journey:

Prepared to offer encouragement to a WYCWYCer who's struggling.

Prepared to help brainstorm ideas for a community member who has reached a roadblock.

Prepared to celebrate the achievements of others as if they were your own.

At the end of the day, being prepared comes down to finding more opportunities, supporting the community, and making fewer excuses.

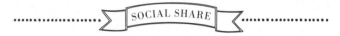

SOCIAL SHARE

Create a Pinterest board specifically for pinning and sharing fun ways to stay prepared. Invite other wycwycers to contribute as well. #wycwyc

BOOKEND YOUR DAY

● ●

IT'S HARD ENOUGH DETERMINING WHAT OUR
healthy living goals are and creating a routine that fits those goals
can feel overwhelming. In a *perfect* world we would have time for
everything we wanted and needed to
do, and our healthy-living plans would
effortlessly integrate into our consistent
daily routines.

> Routine is liberating, it
> makes you feel in control.
>
> –*Carol Shields*,
> author of
> *The Republic of Love*
>
> #wycwyc

Do we even need to say it? This is *not*
happening. There is no perfect world.

However, crafting a certain kind of
sustainable routine for our lives is a powerful means of providing at least some
structure—and sanity!—to our days.
And since we have the least control over the middle (work portion)
of our day, we like to focus on the beginnings and the ends of our
days, which we call "bookends." For example:

* Every morning, do thirty squats or jumps or skips while getting ready for work.

* Every evening, have a music-blaring, calorie-torching cleanup dance party.

Of course, what activities you can fit in will vary, and it's important to be consistently flexible. But we've found that bookending our days with even the briefest of healthy-living routines does wonders to keep our heads in the WYCWYC game. When we start out our day with an activity that furthers our goals—even if it's a short one—and then end our day on a positive note, it's far easier to sustain our long-term plans. We're also more likely to feel proud that we inched ourselves closer to our goals.

Creating bookend routines mentally sets us up for success. So instead of waking up wondering, "How on earth am I going to get everything done today?" we get out of bed thinking, "If nothing else, at least I will {insert your bookend habit here}."

Bookending can also help us feel we haven't failed just because we didn't complete everything on the day's to-do list. Instead, we're reminded that we're *succeeding*, because we're doing WHAT WE CAN WHEN WE CAN to reach our goals. Through bookending, we at least know we'll begin and end our days mindfully striving in the right direction.

It's really pretty simple: In the morning, set the tone for the day. At night, set yourself up for success tomorrow. At the very least, you'll always have your bookends.

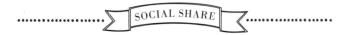

SOCIAL SHARE

Ask others in the WYCWYC community to share their bookend activities—and share yours! You may just inspire someone else to start a new healthy habit! #wycwyc

PLAY!

• •

AS ADULTS WE HEAR THE WORD "PLAY" AND immediately associate it with children. Children play. Adults relax, rejuvenate, have fun, recharge, enjoy downtime, unwind, and take breaks. But rarely do we say, "Let's play!"

> And forget not that the earth delights to feel your bare feet and the winds long to play with your hair.
>
> – *Kahlil Gibran*
>
> #wycwyc

It's time to reclaim the greatest activity of all. Why do we let kids have all the fun? What's not to be gained from seizing a few moments to frolic?

Making time for play gives us the freedom to learn, create, socialize, challenge ourselves, and lose all track of time as we immerse in something that is purely joyful. When was the last time you prioritized something that potent? When was the last time you did *anything* simply for the sheer fun of the activity?

Now that you think about it, don't you miss it?

Play is an important aspect of both our physical health and our mental vibrancy. And fortunately, there are many different ways to play. Consider this vast array of "playportunities":

- ★ Badminton
- ★ Baseball
- ★ Basketball
- ★ Catch
- ★ Croquet
- ★ Dodgeball
- ★ Four square
- ★ Hockey
- ★ Hopscotch
- ★ Horseshoes
- ★ Hula hoop
- ★ Jump rope
- ★ Jumping jacks
- ★ Kickball
- ★ Lacrosse
- ★ Leapfrog
- ★ Miniature golf
- ★ Monkey bars
- ★ Obstacle courses
- ★ Pogo stick
- ★ Red Light, Green Light
- ★ Red Rover
- ★ Shuffleboard
- ★ Skip-It
- ★ Snowball/water gun fights
- ★ Soccer
- ★ Softball
- ★ Squash
- ★ Stilts
- ★ Swings
- ★ Tag
- ★ Tennis
- ★ Tetherball
- ★ Twister

There's also:

- ★ Bike riding
- ★ Bowling
- ★ Climbing
- ★ Dancing
- ★ Ice skating
- ★ Juggling
- ★ Roller skating
- ★ Skateboarding
- ★ Skipping
- ★ Swimming
- ★ Trampoline jumping
- ★ Unicycling

PLAY!

What did we miss? We know you can think of more! The important thing is to find the games you love to play, and to play them WHEN YOU CAN, both for health and for fun. When you see how much activity play can bring to your day, you'll start to wonder why we ever *work* out at all when there are so many opportunities to *play* out! Here are a few ways you can start integrating play into your day:

* Race your kids to the car to see who gets there first.

* See how far you can run along a curb without falling off. Can you make it to the end?

* Grab the kids in the neighborhood for an outside game of Hide-and-Seek.

* Join an after-work softball team.

* Challenge your partner to a tennis match for your next date.

* Invent your own game!

Keep in mind, this is not just about the physical activity. WYCWYC living isn't strictly about goal achievement; it's about moving, engaging, and finding balance. And that's what play is all about too.

Hop. Skip. Jump. Dance. Play.

It all counts.

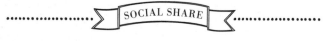

> SOCIAL SHARE

Do a little research online or ask the WYCWYC community if there are any organized games in your neighborhood. If not, why not start your own? #wycwyc

DAILY CONSIDERATIONS

27

MOVE THROUGHOUT YOUR DAY

• •

SO OFTEN PEOPLE EQUATE EXERCISE WITH A preset, preplanned time to "work out." More than that, many of us tend to think "working out" only happens inside some large, intimidating, franchised gym.

Now, we're guessing that you've already gleaned that every single move we make counts.

Not only does each move count all those seemingly small movements add up to create an activity-filled day.

And really, what do all those gym-goers head to the gym to do?

Move.

> I move, therefore I am.
> – Haruki Murakami
>
> #wycwyc

Most people don't suddenly wake up one morning with a burning desire to go for a run or hit the weights. So, to get things started, we can become more mindful of the movement choices we make throughout the day.

Keeping in mind that there are no right or wrong answers, consider the following:

- When there are stairs next to an escalator, which do you choose?

- Think back to the last hotel you stayed in. Did you even know where the stairs were?

- Do you circle a parking lot looking for the closest spot?

- When was the last time you carried a basket rather than pushing a cart at the grocery store?

- Come autumn, do you grab the leaf blower or get out that trusty rake? (As appropriate for your climate, feel free to consider a snow-clearing version of this question.)

- Do you have a habit of sending coworkers email when you could just walk to their desks?

- Do you multitask while on the phone? If yes, is there any movement involved?

- Do you put off cleaning the house/taking out the trash/weeding your garden?

- When was the last time you grabbed the sponge and hose to wash your car?

Again, this isn't about judging any "I do the lazy one" replies you might have made. We simply wanted to initiate the idea that there are lots of ways to move more throughout the day. Even something as basic as using the manual door when there is an automatic option verges on resistance training.

Heck, even fidgeting burns upward of three hundred calories per day!

All these additional small movements, when layered upon each other on a regular basis, will move you closer to your healthy-living goals. And once you start viewing your day through the wycwyc lens, you'll notice even more ways to infuse movement into your life.

As we've mentioned, movement begets movement. And who knows? All that movement might take you to some unexpected places.

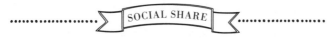

SOCIAL SHARE

Start a twenty-four-hour Twitter challenge and see which of your friends can climb more stairs today! #wycwyc

28

REDUCE
SCREEN TIME

• •

DO YOU KNOW HOW MANY HOURS YOU SPEND
in front of a screen? Two? Four? Eight? Twelve?

These days, much of work, play, and entertainment seems to involve a screen. Worse yet, it involves sitting *passively* in front of that screen.

> We've reached the moment of the perfect storm, when we are more aware of the . . . dangers of hyperconnectivity to technology. We take better care of our smartphones than we do ourselves.
>
> *– Arianna Huffington*
>
> #wycwyc

Take a moment to really think about how much of your day is spent in a state of distraction scrolling through the news, watching a sitcom, or reading Facebook. Now, don't get us wrong: we ourselves couldn't give up Facebook, and we both could be considered TV addicts. But through experience we've learned the value of hitting the Off button from time to time, opening up the space for other things that are important to us.

For example, reducing our screen time overall allows us to

BE MORE PRESENT IN OUR LIVES.

From overly loud commercials and laugh tracks to that all-too-familiar you've-got-mail *ding*, there always seems to be some electronic vying for our attention. But making the conscious choice to put aside our technology for a time offers us an opportunity to be present in a way that's nearly impossible otherwise.

STOP SPECTATING OTHER PEOPLE'S LIVES.

Unplugging also redirects us from being passive observers of other people's lives to more fully live in our own. But there's even more to it than that. Paying close attention to others' experiences makes it all too easy to compare and we might end up thinking theirs is better. When we step away from the highlight reel of other people's lives, we stop comparing, and essentially say: "I am enough. What I do is enough. My experiences are enough." Acknowledging that is vital and lies at the core of the WYCWYC mindset.

KEEP *ALL* LINES OF COMMUNICATION OPEN.

We'd be the first to tell you that social media has been life-changing for us, playing a key role in our successes so far. But we also know it's not technology at the heart of that success, but the human connections and relationships—which technology simply helps us to find and maintain. So, yes, given our modern lives, technology allows us to connect with like-minded people we couldn't otherwise reach. But it's also important not to neglect the more personal means of communication, especially face-to-face time. WYCWYC may be a social media movement, but it's also a mindset, a mantra, and a mission. Screen time can come later.

SEE ALL THE OPPORTUNITIES AROUND US.

Some of the simplest ways to hop on the WYCWYC bandwagon start with closing your laptop, powering down your tablet, silencing your phone, and turning off the television. Just by hitting that Off button, you'll find a number of wycwyc opportunities revealing themselves:

* A backyard game of catch

* Reading

* Going to the park

* Stretching

* Taking a walk with a friend

* Writing in your journal

* Organizing your junk drawer

* Cooking a healthy meal with the family

Of course we could go on and on. The point is for you to consider what you'd be able to do with that extra time. Not to mention that all these suggestions call for active *engagement* rather than passive consumption. That's what we love most about reducing screen time. Being truly engaged reminds us of what's really important in our lives, what brings us joy.

Remember, we're not suggesting you shed the screens entirely. Just mix it up a bit! Get more engaged: turn on the music, go outside, call an old friend while dinner is cooking. Keep all lines of communication open, the more personal the better.

> SOCIAL SHARE

Announce to the wycwyc community that you're having a screen-free day—and then log off! It can be done; prove it! #wycwyc

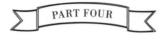

PART FOUR

FOOD FOR THOUGHT

29

CONSUME CONSCIOUSLY

• •

WE WOULD LOVE TO ERADICATE THE WORD "diet" from our vocabulary—at least in the sense of stringently restricting certain foods for a specific amount of time in order to reach a particular number on the scale or fit into what we think is the perfect size.

> He showed the words "chocolate cake" to a group of Americans and recorded their word associations. "Guilt" was the top response. If that strikes you as unexceptional, consider the response of French eaters to the same prompt: "celebration."
>
> – *Michael Pollan*
>
> #wycwyc

For many, the word "diet" stirs up images of bland salads, boiled chicken, and gallons of cabbage soup—as if the only way to lose weight were to avoid foods from specific groups altogether. Some even go to the extreme of not eating at all.

Do any of these comments sound familiar?

★ "This week I'm skipping all carbs!"

★ "Is it fat-free? I'm on a diet."

★ "Oh, no thank you, I'm only eating yellow vegetables this week."

Dieting not only affects our food choices; it also influences our relationships and bleeds into our social lives. For example:

★ "Sorry, I can't go out tonight. I'm doing a cleanse."

★ "I really don't want to go to Susy's party this weekend. I just started a new diet and I know she'll have cupcakes."

★ "Go without me. I'm low-carbing."

But we don't have to approach the food we consume from a mindset of restriction and avoidance. There is no healthy "on" or "off" when it comes to eating; we can't survive if we don't eat.

So, instead of "dieting," try approaching food choices from a perspective of doing WHAT YOU CAN WHEN YOU CAN. That means you take each day, and each meal, as it comes—and do so consciously.

With each food choice, consider its impact on whatever goals you have—say, weight loss, or lower cholesterol, or more fiber—and whether that choice would bring you closer to or further from your goals. Sometimes you'll feel inclined toward a choice that moves you a bit further from your goals, and that's okay. We're here to tell you these choices *can* be made without guilt or shame.

Of course, we can't eat anything we want whenever we want (who else would live off coffee and doughnuts?). But there's no need to feel shame or guilt about indulging.

All of our food choices really do boil down to the notion of *balance*. Consider these scenarios . . .

WHAT'S THE SITUATION:
You really want a breakfast of eggs, bacon, and hashbrowns at your favorite diner.

WHAT YOU CAN DO ABOUT IT:
Enjoy that! But maybe swap the sunny-side up for an egg white

omelet. Then at lunch opt for a salad with grilled chicken and dressing on the side.

WHAT'S THE SITUATION:
Your birthday wouldn't be your birthday without a big slice of cake.

WHAT YOU CAN DO ABOUT IT:
Savor it and move on!

WHAT'S THE SITUATION:
You're out with friends who like to order lots of appetizers.

WHAT YOU CAN DO ABOUT IT:
Partly share in the appetizer fun, and then choose a lighter dish or even a soup for your entrée.

Consuming consciously is all about making choices: some of them indulgent, some not. By approaching our food from a WYCWYC perspective, we can find the middle ground between the guilt of excess and the deprivation of dieting, and get off the emotional roller coaster many associate with eating.

It's time to *consciously* enjoy the ride.

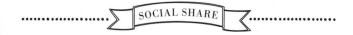

Share a creative shot of your healthy lunch with the community. You never know—you may have a positive influence on someone else's lunch choice! #wycwyc

30

FIND HEALTHY DISTRACTIONS

• •

THERE'S AN OLD DIETING TIP THAT RECOM-
mends we brush our teeth right after dinner so that nothing will
taste good afterward. This approach may work for you, but we've
found we need more than toothpaste in our arsenal when we're
struggling with bad snacking habits. While
we can't promise you'll be motivated all
the time, we can help you arm yourself
with a set of healthy distractions for when
your inspiration wanes.

Part of the WYCWYC life is about stopping
yourself from going down a path that may
take you further away from your goals.

Our goal here is to facilitate your discov-
ery of healthy ways to make yourself feel

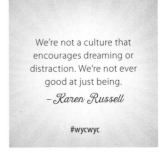

We're not a culture that
encourages dreaming or
distraction. We're not ever
good at just being.

– *Karen Russell*

#wycwyc

taken care of and nurtured, and protected from your own inclina-
tions to stray from what you really want. These distractions can be
readily available and inexpensive, and they don't even have to edge
you closer to your goals.

Create a healthy roadblock.

••••••••●•••••••••

Did you get that? *They don't have to edge you closer to your goals*.

This may seem contradictory to our forward-momentum concept—and of course we want to achieve our goals. But we're here to tell you that sometimes it's important to celebrate the mere fact we haven't taken any steps backward! On some days, the victory is in simply maintaining status quo.

Don't make light of this: the ability to recognize you need a healthy distraction is actually an indication of growth and progress in and of itself. Remember, half the battle in this healthy-living endeavor is recognizing when you're heading down a path that isn't serving you.

Healthy distractions are powerful but uncomplicated. And they can be as simple as texting a friend or cleaning out a drawer. Here are some that work for us:

* Drawing or painting

* Gardening

* Getting a massage or manicure/pedicure

* Journaling

* Reading

* Scrapbooking

* Sewing, Knitting, Crocheting

* Taking a bubble bath

* Taking a nap

* Taking a walk

* Window shopping

- ★ Working puzzles or Sudoku

- ★ Writing a letter

- ★ Calling an old friend

- ★ Reaching out to wycwyc friends on social media

Finding distractions is really just another way of reminding yourself of the activities that bring you joy. When we find pursuits that energize us, the activity becomes less about forcing ourselves to find distractions and more about doing something we love.

$$\text{SOCIAL SHARE}$$

Share a way you positively distracted yourself today. You may inspire someone who is also struggling. #wycwyc

31

ADD IN!

• •

MANY PEOPLE EQUATE HEALTHY LIVING WITH deprivation and hard work, seeing it as all about *can't*: What you can't have. What you can't do. What you can't enjoy.

Not us wycwycers!

On our healthy-living journeys we choose to focus on the wide variety of things we get to "add in."

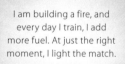

I am building a fire, and every day I train, I add more fuel. At just the right moment, I light the match.

– *Mia Hamm*

#wycwyc

How about adding a new healthy food every day?

Or adding fifty steps to your treadmill time?

Or having an extra glass of water?

You could even schedule yourself an extra fifteen minutes of sleep!

Not only do these additions move you forward; they could also be considered rewards rather than punishments.

Adding in gets our momentum ball rolling in a big way! By reframing the way you think about healthy living—remember how powerful turning your words inside out can be?—and focusing on fun additions instead of perceived sacrifices, you set yourself up for success.

The "add-in" concept can be applied to everything—from what you eat to how you move. For example:

* Add in more vegetables to stews and chili

* Add in fruit instead of skipping dessert

* Add in more steps by taking the stairs

* Add in more joy by logging off the computer and playing

* Add in more laughter by engaging with friends

* Add in more space by giving something away

While the rest of the world focuses on what they *can't* have, do WHAT YOU CAN WHEN YOU CAN and add in!

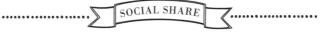

SOCIAL SHARE

Snap a photo celebrating something you added in this week and share it with the community. Ask what add-ins others have discovered too. #wycwyc

32

CHOOSE SMALL

••

EVEN THOUGH WE WYCWYCERS LOVE TO LIVE
large, "small" is one of our favorite words, because it's one of the most
powerful tools in our WYCWYC toolkit. For example:

> Why not do away with
> your super-size options?
> – *Morgan Spurlock*,
> *Super Size Me*
>
> #wycwyc

SMALL STEPS. There's never really anything small when it comes to making healthy
choices. Everything counts. All those shuffles
forward propel us toward success.

SMALL GOALS. Instead of focusing on one
big end goal, we can set ourselves up for success by breaking down larger goals into mini-
goals we can more quickly achieve.

SMALL BITES. If we consume our portions in smaller bites, we'll
have more bites to enjoy.

SMALL PLATES. A smaller portion served on a smaller plate can look like more and can satisfy just the same as a "regular" serving.

SMALL PORTIONS. We've found that with smaller portions we're able to fully enjoy and savor our meal—that the smaller portion is in fact perfectly satisfying.

SMALL SHIFTS. Motivation is often a result of many small mental shifts woven together over time. When these incremental shifts are added together, a whole new mindset results.

SMALL CELEBRATIONS. No achievement is too tiny to celebrate. Ever.

This chapter is short for a reason: we've discovered that the power of *small* can apply to all realms of our lives. Sometimes doing WHAT YOU CAN WHEN YOU CAN is as simple as saying, "Small, please."

⟩ SOCIAL SHARE ⟨

Have you wanted to join in the WYCWYC movement online but haven't yet taken the leap? Start small! Flip to the appendix for some ready-made tips or quotes you can tweet or post on Facebook. When you include the #wycwyc hashtag, others can respond and retweet you! #wycwyc

33

SWAP IT OUT!

• •

IN PART THREE: "DAILY CONSIDERATIONS," WE addressed swapping passive pastimes for active activities. The same approach can work with other healthy-living concerns as well.

First, let's consider the large benefit we can glean from small but powerful food swaps:

> We have more possibilities available in each moment than we realize.
>
> – *Thich Nhat Hanh*
>
> #wycwyc

★ Instead of pancake syrup, use fresh crushed fruit or applesauce.

★ Have a favorite dip? Dip carrots instead of tortilla chips.

★ Use lettuce in place of tortillas when making wraps.

★ Use applesauce rather than butter or oil when baking.

★ Sweet potatoes or butternut squash make great fries.

★ Swap in yogurt instead of mayo or sour cream.

* Replace salt with herbs.

* Prepare old-fashioned or steel-cut oatmeal instead of processed, sugar-laden cereal.

* Instead of cheese and crackers, have cheese and cucumber slices.

* Swap in mashed avocado for the mayonnaise in your sandwich.

* In place of soda, drink seltzer with a splash of juice.

As you can see, the smallest, simplest swaps can create a big ripple effect for your healthy-eating goals. And the food-swapping possibilities are almost endless!

But it doesn't stop there; the swapping trick can also be applied to life in general. It's an additional way to remind ourselves to remain flexible in the pursuit of our goals. We make plans. We focus on plans. Sometimes we realize that our plans don't quite fit our current needs. So what do we do? We swap!

It's not only okay to swap from time to time, it's also smart. It means you're growing more in tune to what your body needs.

It might look a little something like this:

* Knees bother you after long runs? Try running in the pool instead.

* Feeling uninspired? Swap the boring workouts for fun PLAYouts.

* Too tired to take the kids to the park? How about a board game night?

* Feeling too tired for resistance training? Swap in yoga.

* Too hard of a day to end it vacuuming? How about just tidy up instead?

* Too brain-dead to finish your work report? Take a break and empty your in-box instead.

Swapping isn't always about exchanging the good for the bad. Your day is filled with lots of small decisions. WYCWYC is all about making those decisions consciously—and moving forward.

Don't get stuck. Simply swap it out!

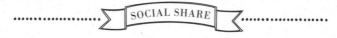

SOCIAL SHARE

Create a Pinterest board of healthy recipe swaps. Invite other community members to pin along with you. #wycwyc

34

SAVOR

• •

HOW OFTEN DO YOU LITERALLY STOP AND
smell the roses, enjoying their scent without rushing past? Or appreciate the color and texture of their petals? The delicate construction
of each flower?

Once your meal is placed before you,
do you dig right in? Or do you pause and
really take it in, relishing the aromas and
colors as much as the flavors? What if you
were to truly taste each unhurried bite?

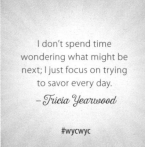

I don't spend time
wondering what might be
next; I just focus on trying
to savor every day.

– Tricia Yearwood

#wycwyc

Though the WHAT YOU CAN WHEN YOU CAN
life is all about snatching all the healthy
opportunities around us, it isn't about
rushing through any of them just to get
them done.

When we eat without thinking about each bite, or when we eat
while watching TV, we don't get as much pleasure from our food—
which can sometimes make us want to eat more than we need. And
besides, food is so great; why would we want to do it unconsciously?

It so happens that when we stop eating mindlessly, choosing instead to slow down and savor what we're "consuming" —whether that be a movie or M&M's—we actually increase our happiness levels.

And we are all about happy!

Savoring is about stretching and prolonging anything that brings us joy. While this may be different for each of us, there's no debating the benefits: slowing down reduces our stress and frees us up to focus on things that are important to us.

And from food to fitness, we have lots of opportunities to savor.

SAVOR INTERACTIONS. When you're with others, truly be with them. Be present. Don't let the day's distractions intrude on your conversations. Engage. Listen. Savor your interactions.

SAVOR FOOD. Really look at your food as you eat it. Pay attention to its tastes, aromas, and textures. This applies as much to a beautiful restaurant meal as it does to your midafternoon snack. Savor the process of fueling your body. And when you indulge, savor the indulgence!

SAVOR TIME. We can make more of most things: money, food, even friends. On the other hand, time, one of our most precious resources, is also very limited. Become more aware of how you spend your time. Prioritize what's truly important, and savor every moment you can.

SAVOR FITNESS. Even if exercise isn't your passion, work to find pleasure in and appreciation of how your body feels during and after activity. The human body is a true marvel—don't take it for granted! Revel in the movement you're capable of; allow yourself a sense of accomplishment for what your body can achieve. Learn to savor movement and love your body for what it can do.

Though the WYCWYC mindset encourages determination in reaching our goals, it doesn't do so to the detriment of living in the now. Savor life now. Don't let your focus on where you want to be distract you from what you have now. Simply savor the process of getting there.

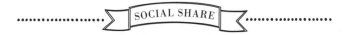

SOCIAL SHARE

Share with the community a photo of a moment you've savored that you previously would have rushed past. Celebrate it! #wycwyc

35

HAVE "TRIED & TRUES"

• •

WE WYCWYCERS BELIEVE IN LIVING A CON-
scious life. We applaud logging off the screen, getting out in the
world, and engaging.

> Technique is what you
> fall back on when you run
> out of inspiration.
> – *Rudolf Nureyev*
>
> #wycwyc

We're empowered! We're mindful and
aware! We're present and in charge!

Until we aren't.

We're human. And sometimes life is
just crazy, and we need a safety net to
fall back on.

This is just another iteration of being
prepared. Given that we know how
effectively life can blindside us sometimes, we've prepared a safety net for
just those times to help us get back on our feet. This net includes
people we know we can rely on, movement options we know keep
us energized, and easy foods we know will nourish our bodies.
Essentially, we've woven into our safety net our "tried & trues."

Tried & trues are wonderfully consistent, reliable, and predictable.

Whether it's the neighbor you can always turn to or that healthy dish from your favorite restaurant, tried & trues are our trustworthy companions on the journey toward our goals. They provide easy solutions for those times when we're not up to making healthy-living choices.

For example, let's say you've had a long day at work. You're exhausted. You're stuck in a traffic jam. You're thinking, "What the heck will I do for dinner?!"

Now, if you hadn't yet considered your tried & trues, then you might find your easiest dinner option is not a healthy one. But if you've already identified your reliable options, then you might realize the following . . .

OPTION 1:
"I'll just swing by the Foodery and grab their great salad."

OPTION 2:
"We've got those frozen leftovers of that new pasta dish we made; I'll pop that in the microwave."

OPTION 3:
"I'll text the sitter to see what she and the kids are having. She's the queen of healthy eating."

When you have your tried & trues worked out in advance, you've set yourself up for success for even the toughest days. So, rather than grappling in the exhausted moment, rather than making excuses, you have ready-made answers.

Of course, tried & trues are different for everyone, so you'll want to contemplate what would work for you *before* the next time you're too exhausted to think. Following are a few areas where tried & trues can be particularly helpful:

★ Research what healthy meal options you have near work, near home, and along your commute in between.

- ★ Keep ingredients on hand and recipes at the ready for a few quick, healthy meals.

- ★ Work up several different exercise options that can work for different windows of time.

- ★ Have healthy "emergency" snacks in the pantry for those munchatastic nights.

It's unrealistic to think we can always be hypervigilant about our healthy-living goals. Part of doing WHAT YOU CAN WHEN YOU CAN to achieve those goals is identifying for yourself reliable options you can fall back on when needed: unique "go-tos" that can carry you through those times you have no brain cells to spare.

Life really is a marathon. Tried & trues are your water stations.

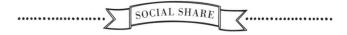

· SOCIAL SHARE ·

Come up with at least one tried & true for yourself from the list above. Then share with the community, and ask others about their picks. #wycwyc

36

HAVE IT YOUR WAY

● ●

"HAVE IT YOUR WAY . . ." A CERTAIN FAST FOOD
chain chimed for forty years.

This slogan got us to thinking. What is it about *specifying* what we
want, even when we're paying someone
else to prepare our meal? Why are some of
us hesitant to state our preferences?

Are we worried the servers will consider
us high-maintenance? Or that our dining
companions will judge us? Are we afraid
we'll be an inconvenience?

Or do we not even realize asking for
what we want is an option?

That certainly was the case for us. We
suffered through meals we would have enjoyed but for a simple
change, like no mayo, or sauce on the side. Looking back from our
current vantage point, it all seems so obvious, but at the time we
didn't have the confidence to ask for *our way*.

It can be challenging at first. There's a certain level of boldness

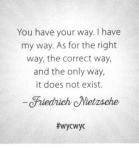

You have your way. I have
my way. As for the right
way, the correct way,
and the only way,
it does not exist.

–*Friedrich Nietzsche*

#wycwyc

required to specify how you want your food prepared, what you'd like alongside, and what you'd like left out altogether. But it's worth it.

This is about building your confidence, and it concerns much more than just healthy eating. Given the ripple effect any WYCWYC actions can make on our lives in general, being self-assured enough to request that your sandwich not have mayo isn't just about one lunch. It builds your confidence toward requesting something bigger, like your boss's permission to take an earlier lunch hour so you can regularly make that yoga class at the gym.

Confidence is an important aspect of the WYCWYC life. You need this confidence not only to ask for the support you require to succeed but also to make requests that help you achieve the goals you've set for yourself.

Confidence really is like a muscle. The more we work it, the stronger it gets—and the easier it becomes to do WHAT WE CAN WHEN WE CAN with our lives.

Be confident. Have it your way.

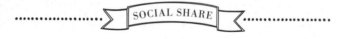

SOCIAL SHARE

Snap a photo of a meal you had your way and share it with the community. #wycwyc

37

CURB YOUR TEMPTATIONS

• •

TEMPTATIONS. WE'RE SURROUNDED BY THINGS that distract us from accomplishing our goals, and we all have our personal vices: food, the couch, the phone, the Internet with its vast array of cute cat videos and endless trivial facts.

By now you'll likely have realized we're not fans of strict rules and deprivation. So that means we believe in occasional indulgences, which can include eating chocolate caramel torte supreme while watching feline hijinks on YouTube.

(But they're so darn cute!)

Yes, they are, but that doesn't mean we

> 'Tis one thing to
> be tempted, another
> thing to fall.
>
> –*William Shakespeare,*
> *Measure for Measure*
>
> #wycwyc

can give in to temptation *all* the time, or we'd never get anything done. So that means we have to find ways to keep the upper hand. From our own experience, we've concluded we can best control temptations by controlling our environment. For example . . .

WHAT'S THE SITUATION:

Let's say you have an ice cream problem. And by "problem" we mean if it's in the house, it's all you think about until the container is empty. (And don't even mention those little mini Häagen-Dazs containers, 'cause they don't cut it.)

WHAT YOU CAN DO ABOUT IT:

Don't keep ice cream in the house! This isn't to say you can never enjoy this creamy delicacy. Just make it less ready at hand. Having to get in the car and drive to Cold Stone Creamery may not always stave off your ice cream imperative, but it will ensure you savor it more than you would in front of the TV.

WHAT'S THE SITUATION:

You'd love to exercise first thing in the morning, but you too easily get sucked into the news report and your in-box.

WHAT YOU CAN DO ABOUT IT:

Don't turn on or look at any electronic device—not even for a moment—until *after* your workout or run. That way you'll have reserved your morning's first activity for yourself only, before you attend to the needs and lives of others.

Since your temptations are individually yours, only you will know how to control them. The WYCWYC lifestyle is all about trusting yourself enough to know when you can't trust yourself at all—and having a plan in place to help you get through it.

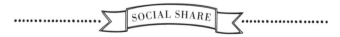

························⟫ SOCIAL SHARE ⟪························

Have you recently resisted a temptation? Share your success story with the community. You never know whom you'll inspire! #wycwyc

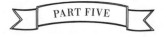
PART FIVE

TRICKS OF
THE TRADE

38

DECLUTTER

· ·

CLUTTER AFFECTS MORE THAN JUST THE cleanliness of our homes—it affects our moods too. And while supposedly there are those who know in *exactly* which pile everything is, that method can't work in a multi-occupant household.

For the rest of us, being surrounded by piles and stacks of stuff is depleting. It can make us feel unproductive, even lazy, reminding us of all the stuff we're just not ready to tackle.

Now we're not suggesting we all have to be Tidy Tessies. We're just saying that keeping the clutter from encroaching on our mental and physical well-being is key to a healthy lifestyle.

If you're really up to it, it can be life-changing to set up an organizational system in your home where "everything has a place and everything's in its place." If you're up to making that happen, more power to you.

> The more I examine the issue of clutter, the more effort I put into combating it, because it really does act as a weight.
>
> –*Gretchen Rubin*,
> author of
> *The Happiness Project*
>
> #wycwyc

Until that day comes, here are a few ways to do WHAT YOU CAN WHEN YOU CAN to reduce the risk of suffocating under a pile of tax receipts, magazines, charity appeals, and take-out menus.

DO HALF! Who says you have to clean everything all at once? Clear off half your desk, sort half your mail, tidy half the family room.

TOUCH IT ONCE. It's so tempting to toss the mail in a pile to deal with later. But sometimes that means you pick up the same envelope, letter, or bill more than once just to figure out what task it demands. Instead, immediately recycle the junk. Then jot on each other piece whatever it needs: "pay," "reply," "cancel," "file"—you get the idea.

THINK TWICE. Make sure you're positive you want or need something before bringing it into the house.

TRADE OFF. Following on that last one: for every new item that comes in the front door, what if another item were to go out the back?

DONATE! "Rehome" the stuff you don't need; many charities, food banks, even animal shelters will welcome your donated items. Plus, think about it: declutter *and* help others? It's a win-win!

ENLIST A FRIEND. Decluttering alone is boring, and it's all too easy to lie to ourselves about what we "need." Invite an honest friend to keep you company and provide feedback as you sort.

BOX UP THE "UNDECIDEDS." But what about those things you *think* you need to keep? How about stashing them in a box stamped with the date? Then, say, a year later, revisit the box. If you haven't missed something in it, you clearly don't need it!

GOOD ENOUGH IS PLENTY. The name of the game here is progress, not perfection. Who really has a perpetually perfect pantry? A continually decluttered closet? The goal is no longer to feel trapped by your stuff. So just chip away at it. Then, once you've uncovered a portion of your desk and recovered a sense of freedom, you can move on with your day.

Decluttering is a lot like getting healthy. It's all about making personal change and shifting your mindset from "ugh!" mode into WHAT YOU CAN WHEN YOU CAN mode. And once your organizational skills start taking shape, you'll instinctively do tomorrow what you have to make an effort to do today.

And you'll have the sorta, almost, definitely, beautifully half-cleaned home to prove it.

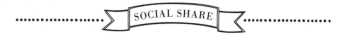

•••••••••••••••••••• ▷ SOCIAL SHARE ◁ ••••••••••••••••••••

Choose something you want to declutter, big or small, and snap a "before" picture. Then, declutter away, celebrating your handiwork with an "after" photo. Share both with the community! #wycwyc

39

HYDRATE HAPPILY

• •

TO US, HYDRATING IS AS WYCWYC AS YOU CAN GET.

One week, "experts" tell us how much water we need, and when we set down our empty glass we pat ourselves on the back. Then the next month different "experts" inform us we're moments away from dehydration.

Since no one can agree on how much water we need each day, we're content to drink WHAT WE CAN WHEN WE CAN and leave it at that.

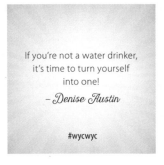

If you're not a water drinker, it's time to turn yourself into one!

– Denise Austin

#wycwyc

Besides, what's wrong with letting thirst be our guide?

In our personal experience, water increases our energy and just makes us feel better. We just don't fret over amounts. So if drinking water doesn't come naturally to you, consider these tips for increased hydration:

* Match your soda or juice intake glass for glass with water.

* Consume water-laden foods like grapes and grapefruit, melons, cucumbers, lettuce, tomatoes, and, of course, watermelon!

* Invest in a fun water bottle, keep it handy, and sip throughout the day.

* Disguise your water. Add fresh or frozen fruit, cucumbers, lemon juice—even carbonation. No one says you can't dress it up. Just drink it.

* Make healthy homemade popsicles!

We've got another "beget" for you: hydration begets hydration. We've found that the more water we ingest, the more our body craves it. As a result, we find ourselves seeking out even more opportunities to hydrate happily.

Cheers!

····················· 〉[SOCIAL SHARE]〈 ·····················

Search the #wycwyc hashtag and see if anyone in the community has started a hydration challenge. If no one has, launch your own! #wycwyc

40

CHILL OUT!

• •

IT'S TIME TO BECOME A WYCWYC HIPPY, SO
put on your bell-bottoms and don your love beads. Why? Because
then you'll be ready for some ace WYCWYC
advice: don't freak out—chill out!

There's no need to freak out about anything. Just take things as they come.

That means:

> Happiness is in the
> doing, not in getting
> what you want.
>
> – *Ethan Hawke*
> in *Before Sunset*
>
> #wycwyc

* Don't freak out about the scale.

* Don't freak out about missing dance class.

* Don't freak out that you ate that cupcake.

* Don't freak out if you ran slower than you did last week.

* Don't freak out about your hectic schedule.

* Don't freak out that your pants are getting snug.

* Don't freak out about the dessert tray they just rolled toward you.

* Don't freak out about that bad photo-tag of you on Facebook.

* And, whatever you do, don't freak out that your workout pants don't match your tank top!

Are you laughing now? Good.

Laughter is a sign that you're relaxing, and that's what we want.

For some of us, this may mean taking deep breaths and accepting our blunders and shortcomings. For others, it may be actively seeking Zen, be that through meditation or time spent with friends. The point is to recognize that doing WHAT YOU CAN WHEN YOU CAN is enough.

The people who are the most successful in life are those who can relax and enjoy the path they travel in pursuit of their goals. Sure, we feel the pressure to achieve, and nothing beats the feeling of pride in a job well done. But we have to take things in stride along the way, because, really, there is no finish line, which means that "along the way" is going to last a long, long time. Too long to come unglued at every turn.

For us personally, what held us back the most was self-induced pressure, stress, and fear. Instead of calmly assessing a bad day or not-so-ideal situation and making a smart WYCWYC decision to get back on track, we'd become frenzied and frazzled, sometimes giving up on things that were really important to us.

But we've learned to chill out since then. We've seen the unnecessary pain and futility of our worried ways and now fall back on the WYCWYC approach to carry us through those stressful times.

When you're regularly doing WHAT YOU CAN WHEN YOU CAN, you can trust yourself to do your best and keep moving forward, one composed step at a time.

Chill out. Let go. Move forward.

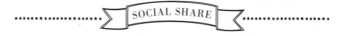

No share this time—just chill. Can you dig it? #wycwyc #peace

41

MEDITATE

• •

Meditation is plotted and planned.
Meditation demands solitude and vast amounts of
    uninterrupted silence.
People who meditate are highly focused and calm.
People who meditate are crunchy granola.

DID YOU AGREE WITH ANY OF THE ABOVE? DO
these descriptions capture your concept of meditation?

We felt the same way . . . until we realized we had it all wrong.
Here's a much better definition, one that
will reveal just how wycwyc meditating
can be:

If you're breathing, you're meditating.

That's it. Stop, notice your breath, and
breathe again. There, that's meditating. You
don't need a local Zen center; you don't

> People think meditation is
> a huge undertaking. Don't
> think of it like that.
>
> – *Deepak Chopra*
>
> #wycwyc

even need a meditation cushion. All you need is to focus on your breath as you inhale, and focus on your breath as you exhale.

Some people like to think "*inhale*" as they breathe in, "*exhale*" as they breathe out. Some like to count: in for four, out for six. Some think "*calm*" or "*relax*." Find what works for you.

It's true that some people meditate for long periods of time. That's because the longer you do it, the more relaxed you feel. And some come to crave that relaxation. But that doesn't mean you have to. Start small. Find your own way.

Once we shifted our concept of what meditation can be, we were able to create an approach that worked for us, one that allows us to reap the multiple benefits of quiet rumination. We de-stress, defuse, and reset ourselves just by consciously, mindfully breathing in and out.

Part of our approach is that you don't have to keep completely still, doing nothing but breathing. You can combine your focused breathing with another activity. Simply take a mindful walk, focusing on each step, each breath.

But the options don't stop there. What about all those times throughout your day when you happen to find yourself alone?

For example, your weekly grocery shopping may have become routine. How about taking those moments to soothe your thoughts before returning to your day?

Or, instead of stressing about the upcoming week while washing up after dinner, you could turn the "monotony" of those stacks of dirty dishes into a meditation of soap bubbles, focusing on each scrub and swipe and rinse.

Then, while you're chopping piles of veggies for tomorrow's lunch, concentrate on the movement, the sound, the aromas, the repetitive *chop* now a centering mantra.

Just as we've described before, the more we seek, the more we find. And the more we've transformed seemingly mindless tasks into moments of breathing awareness and self-care, the more they have become a valuable part of our daily lives. Anytime we can momentarily tune inward and find some calm moves us toward our healthy-living goals.

So take a moment, right this moment, and pause and redirect your mind to your breath.

You've just snagged a moment of meditation, no props, music, or darkened room required.

Relax.

Ease into it.

Allow yourself to discover, as we have, that you already know how to meditate. You do have the time to weave it into your day.

You're already doing it.

> SOCIAL SHARE

What repetitive—even boring—task is on your priority list today? Share with the community how you will transform that chore into a meditation. #wycwyc

42

LAUGH

• •

WHEN WAS THE LAST TIME YOU EXPERIENCED a real, deep-from-the-belly, can't-quite-catch-your-breath, tears-streaming-down-your-face laugh? Can you remember?

The trouble is, in our society laughter can be seen as frivolous, juvenile, and laugh*ers* can be seen as no one to take seriously. So many of us work to present ourselves to the world as no-nonsense, highly focused *grown-ups*.

> Laugh. Laugh as much as you can. Laugh until you cry. Cry until you laugh. Keep doing it even if people are passing you on the street saying, "I can't tell if that person is laughing or crying, but either way they seem crazy, let's walk faster."
>
> –*Ellen DeGeneres*
>
> #wycwyc

Not only do we WYCWYC types believe life is too short not to stop and seek the guffaws; we also are aware of the myriad benefits of chortling.

Let's break it down.

LAUGHING IS A FULL-BODY EXERCISE. Laughing burns calories, elevates heart rate, and even engages the abs!

LAUGHING IS NATURE'S ANTIDEPRESSANT. Laughter releases feel-good chemicals like dopamine in the brain.

LAUGHING INCREASES OUR IMMUNITY. These effects can last from thirty to sixty minutes afterward.

LAUGHING IS FREEING. Don't take life or yourself too seriously. Chill. The times we let ourselves go and truly live often become the moments we savor the most.

When it comes down to it, joy is so effective at bringing us closer to our healthy-living goals, it really could be a goal in and of itself! Now, how can you get more joyful laughter in your life? You've likely already identified your favorite sitcoms, and perhaps regularly seek out funny movies not to mention blooper reels on YouTube. But what about seeing stand-up comedy at a club? Hosting a game night with friends? Push yourself out of your comfort zone and have some fun! Sing karaoke, dance in the rain, get muddy with your kids, try to limbo, roller skate—it all adds up.

Even the less easily amused among us can benefit. Studies show that our brains cannot discern the difference between spontaneous laughter and manufactured giggles. Force a smile, and the brain surmises you must be feeling happy. You can literally fake it 'til you make it, laughter-style!

Our moods are also highly influenced by those around us. So seek out those Jovial Jodys and Hilarious Hals. By keeping you in stitches, these friends are helping move you toward your healthy-living goals.

Laughter is no laughing matter. Relish what you can.

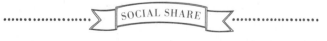

SOCIAL SHARE

Give the wycwyc community a grin today and tell a joke or a funny story about yourself. Everyone loves a smile break! #wycwyc

43

EVEN IF YOU CAN, DON'T!

• •

WE'D LIKE TO EXPLORE ANOTHER ANGLE OF the wycwyc philosophy. Up until now we've been discussing the ins and outs of *doing* what you can to pursue your goals. But sometimes the best way to do that is to *not do* something that intrudes upon or interrupts you in the moment, to essentially prioritize what you're already doing and not give in to the intrusion.

> Just because you can
> Doesn't mean you should
> If it don't do nobody
> Don't do nobody no good.
>
> *– Catherine Russell,*
> jazz and blues singer
>
> #wycwyc

Let's say you're having a hectic day. The computer's been pinging all afternoon. You're trying to tidy up before your book club meeting tonight. Piles of dirty dishes await you in the sink. The kids are whiny. The dog won't stop barking. The car decided to get a flat tire. Oh! and you forgot to defrost something for dinner. (Classic "Calgon, take me away" scenario.)

Then you hear your phone buzz.

What do you do?

We get addicted to those rings and pings; it's easy to feel compelled to answer right away, either because we think we "should" or because it just seems easier to get it over with. *But we don't have to.* Sometimes just because we can doesn't mean we should. Instead, we:

★ Don't read email until we are ready to give it the attention it demands and reply. It's only going to be an addition to our day's already too long to-do list.

★ Don't pick up the phone if we are currently focusing on another priority in our life. It may not be worth the distraction, and it's a disservice to the other person if we can't be present.

★ Don't hop on the latest diet craze just because everyone else is. Sure, we could, but we choose not to. We are the experts of us.

★ Don't reply to a text immediately if we are chatting in a face-to-face conversation. Remain present with the person at hand and respond later. Isn't that the beauty of technology?

★ Don't continue to force ourselves to attend a fitness class we have no passion for. It may be convenient, but if it doesn't light our fitness spark, we move on. We spend our time more wisely on things that bring us joy.

★ Don't answer the door when we are engaged in monotasking. It's okay to be selfish. If it's important they'll come back.

Although it's true, throughout this book that we've emphasized the benefit of snagging opportunities as they present themselves, it's also true that a good wycwycer knows the difference between an opportunity and a disruption, an interference and a priority.

Here we're emphasizing the *when* of WHAT YOU CAN WHEN YOU CAN. And for the disruptions and interferences, we have a reply: "Not now."

Sometimes you'll feel you can handle anything that comes your way, happily wycwycing your way to your goals, managing all the diversions that present themselves, and balancing your wants and needs like a pro. That's great, and it's certainly true that some people thrive on being on top of many things at once.

But some days you can't. Some days require you to streamline, to monotask, to stay with what you've prioritized. So do that, and let the rest wait their turn.

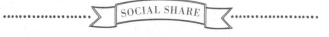

Share a "not now" moment you're especially proud of with the community. We can all use encouragement around being responsibly selfish. #wycwyc

44

PRIORITIZE SLEEP

•••

WE'RE BOMBARDED BY STATISTICS TELLING US how sleep-deprived our culture is and how we need to get more rest. But do we really need the experts to tell us this?

Hey, if you're dancing till the wee hours, we tip our wycwyc hats to you. But the rest of us can't attribute our sleep deprivation to late-night frolicking— we're too busy just trying to squeeze all that needs doing into the time we have, which seems never to be enough. And to compound the issue, when we're not stealing time from sleep by tending to our to-do lists, we steal from sleep *fretting* about those lists.

> It is a common experience that a problem difficult at night is resolved in the morning after the committee of sleep has worked on it.
>
> *–John Steinbeck*
>
> #wycwyc

There's no getting around it: getting enough sleep is essential to living a healthy life. Our bodies and brains require a certain amount of recharging and behind-the-scenes maintenance. When we don't get enough rest, our energy levels are sapped, and we can't function

*Most of us force ourselves to get by
on too few hours of sleep.*

...........•............

optimally. In essence, sleep deprivation sets off a negative momentum that can be difficult to turn around.

Our solution: prioritize sleep, and create an environment that's conducive to high-quality rest.

Now you might imagine this is nearly impossible to achieve, and that we're crazy for even suggesting you try. But we assure you, speaking as two sleep-deprived mamas, that there are a number of approaches to help you get enough shut-eye. For example . . .

LIMIT YOUR CAFFEINE INTAKE AFTER MIDDAY. Caffeine's effects can last from eight to ten hours! Make sure it's not affecting you when you need to get to sleep.

TAKE TIMED CATNAPS IF YOU CAN. The National Sleep Foundation cites twenty- to thirty-minute naps as greatly beneficial in recharging our batteries and productivity.

CREATE A WIND-DOWN ROUTINE. Have nightly patterns that signal to your brain it's time to slow things down. This might include putting your pajamas on thirty minutes early, relaxing with a cup of night-time tea, and practicing a guided meditation just before bed.

SET THE STAGE. Make sure the room is dark and cool. In addition, some sleepers find earplugs, eye masks, and relaxing sounds or white noise helpful in improving the quality and even the quantity of their sleep.

KEEP IT SIMPLE. Ideally, the only things happening in bed would be sex and sleep. If we want our brains not to associate the bedroom with spreadsheets and schedules, we'd be wise to keep our workaday electronics out of the room.

FIGHT THE FRAZZLES. But even if you do ban the gadgets from the sleep chamber, it can still be hard to power down your mind at night. If you keep paper and pencil handy, you can jot down any worries or to-do items for the next day. Getting the worries out of your head and onto the paper can help you get the sleep you need tonight to tend to the items tomorrow.

Of course, none of us is perfect, and these examples in their entirety might seem possible only in a perfect world. All we're saying is that if we prioritize sleep, we'll be better prepared to pursue our healthy-living goals. And how can you acknowledge sleep is a priority? By doing WHAT YOU CAN WHEN YOU CAN to get enough of it.

Turn off the light. Sleep tight.

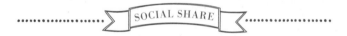

SOCIAL SHARE

Announce you're off to bed, say goodnight to your #wycwyc friends, power down the electronics, and go get some sleep. #wycwyc

MAKE A LIST

• •

WITH ITS LAYERS OF RESPONSIBILITIES—FROM
work to family to even play and prioritizing healthy living—life can
be mentally paralyzing.

> ★ Working late all this week, bills coming due, the kids' game this
> weekend, and the car needs to be serviced . . .

Give me a laundry list and
I'll set it to music.
–*Gioacchino Rossini*

#wycwyc

> ★ We need to plan Cameron's birthday
> party, but how to fit it in with every-
> thing else that needs to get done?

> ★ When the heck will I get to the gro-
> cery store—or even eat, for
> that matter?

In the moments when we feel we have
too much to do and not enough time in
which to do it, we've found the most freeing and fulfilling solution is
also our most plain and simple practical tip: make a list.

Everything feels much more
complicated when it's swirling
around in our heads.

••••••••●●••••••••

Part of the beauty of list-making is simply the act of emptying our heads. The sheer mental jumble of it all can feel weighty and chaotic in our minds, but when jotted down and in front of us, the gotta-dos and don't-forgets are never as large or as impossible as we'd feared.

Lists can be gold for the heavily committed WYCWYCer. On those days when you feel overwhelmed and discouraged, pause, grab paper and pencil or screen and keyboard, and dump the stray to-do items swirling in your brain into a list you can see. This seemingly small WYCWYC strategy is actually really powerful, as it relieves the brain of the stress of keeping tabs on all those details, tasks, and to-dos plaguing you. And downloading all those tasks from your brain can feel like a small accomplishment of its own, which means you're already making progress! Even that alone can be enough to get the ball rolling.

Once you're armed with your list, pick the smallest, easiest item, complete it, and enjoy the satisfaction of crossing it out or checking it off as *done*. Then, repeat! Keep that forward momentum going. We even like to include on our list something we've already completed; anything that gives us the pleasure of crossing off an item can be valuable in propelling us ever forward.

Now, some of you ultra-busy WYCWYCers may disagree—you may insist your head list is better kept in the dark, that it would be ter-rifyingly long if it was visible in front of you. That's okay. We can still promise you one thing: regardless of the length, creating a list frees your mind. You're grabbing a wycwyc opportunity and bringing order to your world.

It releases your mind from all that *remembering* so you can focus on *accomplishing*. Then you are on your way!

List. Complete. Repeat.

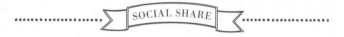

SOCIAL SHARE

Feeling overwhelmed? Take a moment to make a list.
Share two or three items with the wycwyc community that
you plan to do today. Don't forget to ask for words of
encouragement if you need them! #wycwyc

46

SET A TIMER

• •

WE ALL LEAD BUSY LIVES. ALL OF US.

Your busy may look different from my busy, but busy is what we all seem to be.

Busy means we have to prioritize. We have to determine what is most important and achievable in our daily lives, and focus our energy on taking care of those top-tier necessities. We do WHAT WE CAN WHEN WE CAN to accomplish what we are able to.

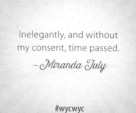

Inelegantly, and without my consent, time passed.

–*Miranda July*

#wycwyc

And that's great! Except when it isn't. Sometimes it's hard convincing ourselves that doing what we can is enough. Sometimes the tasks we *aren't* accomplishing weigh heavily on us. Or worse, sometimes we put them off for being too time-consuming, too complicated, or even too annoying—even if they do actually make our lives easier.

Sound familiar? It's called procrastination.

Thankfully, we've found a way around our procrastination with the use of a tiny, otherwise inconspicuous, handy and helpful little device: a timer!

But first, let's back up a bit. Consider the items on your to-do list that never seem to get done. Tasks such as organizing the garage, decluttering your closet, and cleaning out the pantry. The items that tend to fall under the umbrella of "Someday, when I have a big chunk of time, I'll tackle that."

Now, instead of seeking that elusive stretch of open, empty time—which may never come—break down each task into smaller increments.

WHAT'S THE SITUATION:
You have a ton of laundry to put away before work, but you have to leave in ten minutes.

WHAT YOU CAN DO ABOUT IT:
Set the kitchen timer for five minutes and do as much as you can. Even five minutes will make a noticeable difference.

WHAT'S THE SITUATION:
Your dinner party is tomorrow, and the entire house is a disaster.

WHAT YOU CAN DO ABOUT IT:
Take fifteen minutes before bed to straighten up the dining room. That will leave less to do tomorrow.

Your timer doesn't have to be an actual timepiece—you can let some established intervals set your start and end times for you. Take advantage of the reliable, brief snippets of time offered by television commercials: chop veggies for tomorrow's snack, or see how many items you can fold in 120 seconds. Even the ending beep of the dishwasher or clothes dryer notes the passage of a set increment of time.

There's a lot of fun to be had using these built-in reminders to help us chip away at our to-do list—*go-go-go* style!

What's more, it's remarkable how "allowing" ourselves only a few minutes at a time to focus on a large task actually makes it feel less daunting. At least you know you've started it—and you're proving it's manageable.

If you haven't made the time, and you can't find the time, set the time. *Ding!*

> ## SOCIAL SHARE

Come up with a two-minute exercise routine and share it with the community. Challenge others to join you during the next commercial break! #wycwyc

PART SIX

BEFORE WE
LET YOU GO

47

COMPARE YOURSELF WITH NO ONE

• •

CONSIDER THIS ADAGE: COMPARISON IS THE THIEF of joy.

Okay, point taken. But it's so difficult not to compare ourselves to others; we can't help ourselves. We could be skipping merrily along, doing WHAT WE CAN WHEN WE CAN, feeling fantastic, and then *bam!* We spy seemingly perfect Sarah Somebody, and our chill, confident attitude gets hijacked by feelings of insignificance and inadequacy.

We've been there.

We've both done this even though we knew nothing about Sarah Somebody—her story, her struggles, her dreams, her failings. We've default to assuming *she* had it better—and that we're lesser in comparison.

> Women are so unforgiving of themselves. We don't recognize our own beauty because we're too busy comparing ourselves to other people.
>
> – *Kelly Osbourne*
>
> #wycwyc

After years of struggling with this, we've come to the realization that, no matter how hard we try, we can't stop noticing differences. But it's important to distinguish:

noticing doesn't have to involve *comparing*. We may notice someone is taller, shorter; thicker, smaller; younger, older. Okay, so let's just register the great variety in all of us, from physical traits to experiences. In fact, let's celebrate the differences. Let's also view these differences as just information, and stop the comparison cycle, which helps no one and may harm us all which is no use to anyone.

But it doesn't stop there. What about the comparisons we make the most, without even realizing it: ourselves against ourselves?

Ourselves younger. Ourselves before kids. Ourselves before an injury. Ourselves before we gained weight.

But then again, what's the point of this sort of comparison? How does lamenting the radiant skin and stamina you had twenty years ago help you pursue your goals today? Where is the benefit in comparing a photo from ages ago with the exhausted woman in the mirror? We're basically measuring an apple against an orange, and diminishing our sense of self-value in the process. And besides, that smooth-cheeked woman didn't know half of what you know now! Nor could she do anywhere near what you can do.

So how about doing a few rethinks . . .

WHAT WE DO NOW:
We get down about how, even though we rocked our run yesterday, we had to walk part of it today.

WHAT WE COULD DO INSTEAD:
Celebrate the fact we even got out there! And trust that we'll rock it again.

WHAT WE DO NOW:
Bitch about all those clothes that no longer fit since the kids came along, and how we now wear yoga pants on a daily basis.

WHAT WE COULD DO INSTEAD:
Celebrate the amazing feat of producing life, and applaud our bodies for enduring pregnancy and parenting.

There's a reason why a car's rearview mirrors are tiny, while the windshield is huge. Like driving, WYCWYC is about focusing on the road right in front of you—and keeping at it.

This book isn't called "What I Could When I Could."

It's not titled "What She Can When She Can."

This book is called *What You Can When You Can.*

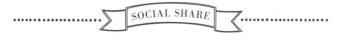

SOCIAL SHARE

Compliment someone you've previously felt competitive with. We are all in this together! #wycwyc

48

MOVE TOWARD MOMENTUM

•••••••••••••••••••••••••••••••••••

AN OBJECT IN MOTION TENDS TO STAY IN
motion. The more momentum an object has, the harder it is to stop it.

No, we aren't giving lessons in physics. We believe these concepts apply to healthy living and goal achievement. These scientific principles tell us how we can create our own personal velocity.

They also teach us that there is a force that can interrupt our momentum and derail our energy: the fear of failure.

Now, a lot of us think of failure as another negative F-word. But we don't have to, nor should we.

Failure isn't scary. Failure is on our side.

All the tips in this book have emerged

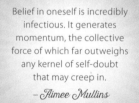

Belief in oneself is incredibly infectious. It generates momentum, the collective force of which far outweighs any kernel of self-doubt that may creep in.

– *Aimee Mullins*

#wycwyc

from our personal experiences, especially our *failures*.

As a result, our definition of failure has drastically changed—and now we embrace it.

Let's say we signed up to run a charity race with friends, but then work got busy, we stopped training, and now we have just three days before the big event.

What do we do?

WHAT WE'D DO BEFORE:
Before, we'd have not participated in the event, and declared ourselves failures. The disappointment in ourselves would have carried over into almost all other areas of our lives.

WHAT WE CAN DO INSTEAD:
Instead, we stay chill, acknowledge we're not perfect, and show up anyway. Even if we walk most of it, who cares? We've maintained our momentum and done what we could!

When we fully adopt the WHAT WE CAN WHEN WE CAN mindset, fear of failure no longer holds power over us—which means it can't stop our momentum.

We accept our imperfections and move forward.

So, now, we're past the starting gate. Let's say we've jogged a bit, skipped a bit, but we're mostly walking. Okay. We're moving, and we're moving toward momentum.

Moving toward momentum means you no longer hinge your happiness or success on achieving a goal—say, crossing the finish line of this particular charity run. Instead, WYCWYCers embrace the *process* without dwelling on how long it may take to reach each milestone.

Sometimes "momentum" will be at a snail's pace. It may feel as if we are hardly making any progress at all. But that's okay. We don't think less of others lagging behind in the race, do we? (Or, ideally we don't.) Other times, we'll have a good rhythm going, with the wind at our back—propelling us swiftly forward.

Either way, our pace won't matter. What matters is that we focus on maintaining momentum.

Remember:

* Awareness begets awareness.

* Confidence begets confidence.

* Encouragement begets encouragement.

* Fearlessness begets fearlessness.

* Happiness begets happiness.

* Healthy eating begets healthy eating.

* Movement begets movement.

The more we do WHAT WE CAN WHEN WE CAN, the more we shift to the WYCWYC mindset and keep moving forward despite the inevitable hiccups, the more effortless it all becomes. We begin to trust in the *potential* of momentum, knowing it will keep us moving toward our goals, toward our successes.

Set yourself in motion and let your momentum go.

Fear is not a strong enough force to stop you anymore.

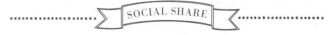

SOCIAL SHARE

Celebrate something you did instead of stopping and losing momentum. The smallest step forward is still a step toward your goals. Celebrate it! #wycwyc

49

PRACTICE PATIENCE

•••

THERE IS ONE FINAL ASPECT TO LIVING THE wycwyc way we haven't yet focused on.

This wasn't an accident. It's a crucial piece of the wycwyc puzzle, an additional tool to go with the other forty-eight in the wycwyc arsenal.

> If you can stick with a goal for long enough, you'll almost always get there eventually. It just takes patience and motivation.
>
> –*Leo Babauta*,
> author of *The Essential Motivation Handbook*
>
> #wycwyc

Patience.

The very notion of baby steps implies persistence, but it's time to address it more specifically.

We need to be patient with the process.

There was a time we just wanted to get there. Nail it. Show up, get the job done, announce our success, and be finished!

Through our personal experience using the wycwyc mentality, we've learned to be patient with the process, to have patience for the full length of the journey. We've realized that big changes don't happen overnight, and healthy living isn't built in a day. This was a struggle for us initially, but now we've come to love the process.

We need to be patient with ourselves.

This one is probably the hardest for many of us, but it's essential that we forgive ourselves at those times when we veer off our healthy living path. And, trust us, we will have many of those times.

Through our WYCWYC experience we've learned to be gentle with ourselves. Over time we've gained confidence in ourselves; we've developed a trust in ourselves that we're always doing the best we can WHEN WE CAN. And that confidence and profound trust we've created only reinforce the message a thousandfold.

We are enough.

Think back to our mention of a baby trying out her first steps. Imagine again the bravery of that small child, that smiling, drooling creature so intent on progressing into life. The few, sweet, awkward steps, the giggly *plop* back on the floor. Treat yourself as you would that child. Be patient with yourself, and celebrate each awkward little step.

We need to be patient with others.

Finally, we must remember to have patience with others as we go on this journey. Even though, along the way, we'll need to turn to others for support, requesting extra encouragement when we don't have enough to offer ourselves, not everyone will understand or support the path we're on. Their priorities may not always align with ours, and that's okay. We carve our own paths; we all have our own goals. Allow others theirs as you request that they allow you yours, as you remain responsibly selfish in pursuing a healthy life.

Be confident. Be calm. Do WHAT YOU CAN WHEN YOU CAN—with patience!

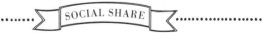

SOCIAL SHARE

Consider a time you've been patient with yourself. Consider a time you've been patient with another. And share one of these patient moments with the community; you'll likely be an inspiration to others. #wycwyc

50

BE A WYCWYC CHAMPION

• •

WHAT YOU CAN WHEN YOU CAN.

#wycwyc (*wick-wick*). Six little letters. One fun hashtag.

Who would have thought it could mean so much?

From adding to quitting, from margins to MUSTurbating: We seized. We savored. We swapped. We laughed. We meditated. We played.

> It takes a lot of courage to show your dreams to someone else.
>
> – *Erma Bombeck*
>
> #wycwyc

Maybe you read this book in one sitting. Or perhaps you flipped through and skipped around, searching for tips that resonated with you. It doesn't matter if you incorporate the tips all at once or add them one by one. What's important is *you're doing it*.

You did what you could when you could when you picked up this book and cracked its cover.

You've already sparked your momentum.

And you're now a wycwycer. A WHAT YOU CAN WHEN YOU CAN ambassador. Someone who knows that small, incremental changes add up over time, and that all combined can produce huge shifts in your life. You know there's no reason to take a seat and wait around for perfect, because it's never coming. And you know that snagging opportunities that inch you closer to your goals are worth the effort, because they keep you moving forward.

This awareness is, in essence, your graduation ceremony. It's your wycwyc commencement in the purest definition of the word—band, tissues, and champagne optional.

But we're not done yet. Just as we encouraged you in Chapter 1 to join a movement, we're now asking you to pay that movement forward.

It's your turn to pass the torch and spread the word. It's your chance to make an impact on others and be a wycwyc champion. That's the bookend to this process.

We invite you to be a wycwyc champion in a fashion that feels natural to you. Maybe you will:

* Talk with a family member about the power of deconvenience, or the benefits of swapping passive for active.

* Confess to a friend how you used to compare yourself with them, until you realized how it affected you and your motivation.

* Tweet to an acquaintance how decluttering your desk helped you focus and find more wycwyc opportunities.

* Strike up a conversation with a stranger in the produce section and share tips about your favorite vegetables.

* Surprise your family with an active Saturday outing. No need to mention you're doing WHAT YOU CAN; just lead by example.

Each time you champion how the wycwyc approach is helping you fulfill your goals, you encourage others in pursuit of theirs. And no matter where you are on your journey, someone else is likely watching you, and inspired by you, admiring your tenacity and wondering how you do it. And each time you champion another's efforts, you also remind yourself how far you've come, how much you know, and how you're still moving forward.

In encouraging others, you empower yourself.

In empowering others, you encourage yourself.

What goes around comes around—and we're all in this together.

The book has ended, yet it's only the beginning.

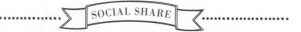
SOCIAL SHARE

Go out and be a WYCWYC champion in the way that feels most comfortable for you. Shout it from the Facebook rafters to all your new #wycwyc friends. Quietly slip a copy of this book to the busy neighbor who asked how you always retain your cool. Start a #wycwyc club, and work through the tips as a group! Do WHAT YOU CAN, do it WHEN YOU CAN, and know we're with you all the way. #wycwyc

THE *SOCIAL* IN SOCIAL MEDIA

• •

EVEN IF DIGITAL COMMUNITIES AND FRIEND- ships are entirely new to you, even if you don't know what a "tweet" is or what it means to update your "status", you don't have to be tech savvy in order to benefit from and enjoy social media. The point is just to find the digital channels that work best for *you*, and we want to help you do that. Here are a few items to consider before you make your first foray into this brave (and beautiful!) new world:

WHAT'S A HASHTAG? Once called the pound sign, #, the hashtag is used in social media to "tag" and filter content by keyword. Using the #wycwyc hashtag allows you to easily find like-minded folks already living the WYCWYC life. You really are never alone.

IF YOU'RE A VISUAL PERSON, a community awaits you on platforms like Pinterest and Instagram. Search for the hashtag #wycwyc to find WYCWYCers sharing photos, offering advice, and building networks. One way to get started is to repost photos by others that you found particularly inspiring, sharing with the community what about them resonated for you. You can also contribute to the community: just tag your images with #wycwyc so others can find you.

IF IT'S WORDS THAT SPEAK TO YOU, your tribe is sharing everything from recipes to success stories on Facebook and Tumblr; and some have their own blogs. "Like" the wycwyc Facebook page (www.facebook.com/hashtag/wycwyc), search the hashtag, and start interacting. Share a little about yourself. Encourage others. Relay a #wycwyc tip that has worked well for you in the past.

IF YOU PREFER TO SHARE ONLY SNIPPETS OF YOUR WYCWYC ACTIVITIES, your people are chatting on Twitter. If you're a newbie, start by searching for #wycwyc and follow a few people who post about their wycwyc life. Start slowly by retweeting some great tips, or jump in and introduce yourself.

ARE YOU MORE OF A SOCIAL MEDIA TRAILBLAZER? As technology shifts and expands, with ever newer social ventures taking hold, the social media landscape will change along with it. Your own online experience will likely evolve as well. Be adventurous; look for wycwycers in all facets of digital life. In addition to the modes mentioned above, there's a wycwyc community exploring ways to connect using Vine and Google+.

For a more comprehensive listing of social media channels, including links, tips, and tricks for searching the #wycwyc hashtag, visit www.wycwyc.com.

And whichever path you choose, remember: the more you interact, the stronger your wycwyc community becomes. We're crazy enough to be on almost every platform. Use the hashtag #wycwyc and come find us!

TWEETABLE #WYCWYC SPARKS

• •

WE'VE GATHERED SOME SAMPLE #WYCWYC sparks to help put you in the mindset of being a social media sharer. Whether you tweet them as tips for others or do them yourself and then celebrate your success with the community, these fun tips are here to inspire and encourage you. They're even short enough for Twitter, as each one has fewer than 140 characters.

RELATIONSHIPS

* A family game night: schedule it now. #wycwyc

* Start more family *convos* with a "Three Things" rule at dinner. Every family member tells at least three things about the day. #wycwyc

* Let your kids do their homework at your desk while you're working. #wycwyc

* Stick a fun note in your child's lunch. #wycwyc

* Surprise your significant other with an unexpected hug. #wycwyc

* Text a friend you haven't had time to connect with. Let her know you're thinking of her. #wycwyc

* Breakfast for dinner is fun. Just sayin'. #wycwyc

* Sunday morning cook-fest. Make chilis, stews, and sauces for the week. #wycwyc

TIME/ORGANIZATION

* Laundry overload? Put a load in when you wake up. Transfer to the dryer before leaving for work. Fold it while watching TV. #wycwyc

* Make an "I Can Delegate" list. Don't worry yet about who. Just realize and list the tasks you don't *need* to do yourself. #wycwyc

* Make household chores family fun time, not watch-Mommy-work time. #wycwyc

* Every night, think about what you'll have for breakfast the next day. Visualize healthy eating being what launches your day. #wycwyc

* Challenge your family to a contest: who can put away the most stray items in ten minutes? Winner gets a one-minute backrub from everyone else. #wycwyc

* Wrap up work five minutes early and straighten your desk. #wycwyc

* Assign ringtones to the important people in your life. If it's them calling, you'll immediately know. #wycwyc

* Clean the shower while taking a shower. #wycwyc

* Consciously "forget" your phone when running errands or when you have work to get done. #wycwyc

* Create multiple email folders. Do a quick triage assessment of and stash all email immediately upon arrival. #wycwyc

* Distracted by social media? Log off. #wycwyc

* Don't attend to an email until you're ready to reply to it. #wycwyc

- ★ Feeling unmotivated to work? Jot down a to-do list and take a break. Come back fresh and ready to check things off when you can. #wycwyc

- ★ Floss, even if one tooth a night. (Just make it a different tooth each night.) #wycwyc

- ★ Garbage night? Take each bag out separately and lap the house before grabbing the next. #wycwyc

- ★ If you haven't used or worn something in over a year, give it away. #wycwyc

- ★ Turn off the TV. You'll be surprised how much more you move without the boob tube distracting you. #wycwyc

- ★ Waiting for dinner to cook? Clean out one drawer or pantry shelf. #wycwyc

- ★ No time to start a family exercise routine? Turn up the music for an informal dance party. #wycwyc

- ★ Make lunches and have coats, shoes, bags, and keys ready by the door the night before. Ten minutes at 8 P.M. saves you twenty in the morning. #wycwyc

EATING

- ★ Instead of a big lunch, arm yourself with healthy snacks and graze through your workday. #wycwyc

- ★ Keep a food journal by snapping a pic on your cell. At the end of the day, review. #wycwyc

- ★ Make a food first-aid kit for your car or purse that's stocked with nonperishable healthy snacks. #wycwyc

- ★ Make your own salad dressings. #wycwyc

- ★ Pair soup with salad instead of a sandwich to avoid the carb overload. #wycwyc

- ★ Pizza night? Order a thin crust with all the veggies. Enjoy. #wycwyc

* Really want that indulgent appetizer? Order it as a meal. #wycwyc

* Really, *really* want pizza? Make one on a tortilla or an English muffin. #wycwyc

* Replace "Extra cheese, please" with "No cheese, I'm good." #wycwyc

* Always drink water at restaurants. Save calories *and* money. #wycwyc

* At least once a month, make a dish using new-to-you produce. #wycwyc

* Craving a comfort food? Indulge with half the portion you'd normally eat. #wycwyc

* Do you *really* need the rice or potato with every meal? Double up on veggies every other day. #wycwyc

* Don't eat anything out of the bag or box. Portion off your one serving. #wycwyc

* Do you tend to finish the kids' meals at the restaurant? Order a soup and salad so you can indulge guilt-free. #wycwyc

* Eat a rainbow of colors as much as possible. #wycwyc

* Eat breakfast. Always. Even if it's just a banana in the car on the way to work. #wycwyc

* End each day with a cup of hot, soothing tea. #wycwyc

* Indulging in a fro-yo visit? Ditch the crumbled candy bars for berries. And maybe add just a few chocolate sprinkles as garnish. #wycwyc

* Give mustard a chance. #wycwyc

* Frozen grapes: try them. #wycwyc

* Had a big lunch? Out to dinner? Send the bread back—immediately. Don't even give yourself time to think about it. #wycwyc

* Hungry? Enjoy a full glass of water before eating. #wycwyc

- ★ When faced with a buffet, use a small plate. Choose lots of green stuff. #wycwyc

- ★ Out for burgers? Try a veggie burger or portabello mushroom burger. #wycwyc

- ★ Swap chocolate chips for cacao nibs. #wycwyc

- ★ Swap frying for grilling, baking, or steaming. #wycwyc

- ★ Eat slowly. Take mini breaks and sip water throughout your meal. #wycwyc

- ★ Tell the waiter you're lactose intolerant and to skip all butter or cream in your entrée. #wycwyc

- ★ Rip off as much as possible of that oversized bun; save your calories for the good stuff. #wycwyc

- ★ The slow cooker is your friend. #wycwyc

- ★ Throw aging fruit in the freezer; make a smoothie the next time you crave ice cream. #wycwyc

- ★ Trim all visible fat from meat before you cook. #wycwyc

- ★ When you cook enough to have leftovers, wrap the extra *before* eating your meal. #wycwyc

- ★ Always order a small. Always. No excuses. #wycwyc

SELF-CARE

- ★ Carry a water bottle everywhere. Hydration rocks. #wycwyc

- ★ Instead of lurking on social media, plan a vacation even if you can't afford it now. #wycwyc

- ★ No matter the season, dab a dollop of sunscreen behind each ear. Let summer scents remind you of stress-free days. #wycwyc

- ★ Pick one grudge you're holding on to or one person you've not forgiven and let it go. #wycwyc

- ★ Prioritize sleep. Even if you can't make *more* time to sleep, create an environment conducive to good-quality sleep. #wycwyc

- ★ Purchase and remember to take multivitamins. Gummies are fun! #wycwyc

- ★ Replace "I should" with "I choose" or "I get to." #wycwyc

- ★ Say "no" more. #wycwyc

- ★ Create a comfort mantra. Pick words or just sounds. Chant when stressed or tempted to mindlessly eat. #wycwyc

- ★ Create a decadence list. Jot down five things that make you feel cared for or nurtured. #wycwyc

- ★ Dance as if no one's watching (even if they are). #wycwyc

- ★ Evoke happy thoughts or memories by looking through a few old photos. It's not a time waster; it's a mood booster. #wycwyc

- ★ Smile at a stranger. You'll be surprised how it brightens your day. #wycwyc

- ★ Stop and smell the roses . . . or cinnamon or vanilla—a scent that transports you to a place you'd like to visit. #wycwyc

- ★ Take five slow, deep, full breaths. #wycwyc

- ★ Focus on your breathing for two minutes (twelve deep breaths). If your thoughts wander, tell them, "Not now," and focus again on your breath. #wycwyc

- ★ Write a letter to yourself. Remind yourself of all the ways you rock. #wycwyc

- ★ Write yourself love notes. Tape one to a mirror. Hide others to be discovered later. Remind yourself why you're wonderful. #wycwyc

- ★ Look ahead on your calendar. Block off self-care time. #wycwyc

- ★ Get into your jammies thirty minutes earlier than usual. #wycwyc

MOVEMENT

- ★ Fidget. Wiggle. Toe tap. Burn extra calories even when you can't fit in a workout. #wycwyc

- ★ Snowstorm? Awesome. Get out there and shovel. Who needs a gym? #wycwyc

- ★ Keep five-pound hand weights behind the couch and sneak some curls while watching the evening news. #wycwyc

- ★ Keep a jump rope in plain sight. When you notice it, see how many jumps you can do without a break. #wycwyc

- ★ Keep an exercise ball in the living room and add in a few crunches while watching TV. #wycwyc

- ★ Lose the remote—deliberately. Keep it away from the couch so you have to get up to change the channel. #wycwyc

- ★ Problem at work? Need to think? Get up and pace. Better yet, take a walk. #wycwyc

- ★ Race the kids: back to the car, between crosswalks, to the mailbox. #wycwyc

- ★ Replace your office chair with an exercise ball. Love the bounce, and your core muscles are feelin' it. #wycwyc

- ★ Jump up and do a touchdown dance for your team when they score. #wycwyc

- ★ Behind on book club reading? Get the audiobook and let someone else do the reading while you take a walk. #wycwyc

- ★ Crank up the music and desk dance. In an office? Solicit your coworkers to join you. #wycwyc

- ★ Do five squats. No, really. Right now. Put the book down and squat. #wycwyc

- ★ Do a downward dog/upward dog yoga sequence before hopping into bed. Your back will thank you. #wycwyc

* Gone are the days of carrying all the groceries in one trip. See how many trips you can make and increase that step count. #wycwyc

* Hold a wall squat while you brush your teeth. Goal: two minutes. #wycwyc

* Schedule your next workout right now. Seriously, open up your calendar and commit. #wycwyc

* Skip the office email to your colleague in the next building; use it as an excuse to take a midday stroll. #wycwyc

* Slept in? Missed your morning workout? Ask a coworker to join you for a lunchtime walk. #wycwyc

* Stand still on the escalator? Never. #wycwyc

* Stuck in traffic? Put on fun music and jitter and dance in your seat. #wycwyc

* Stuck waiting for something? Use that time to work on your balance. Stand on one leg for as long as you can, then switch. #wycwyc

* Waiting for something to heat up in the microwave? Counter push-ups. #wycwyc

* Replace one TV show a day with a game of catch or a walk. #wycwyc

* No more dinner and movie dates. Mix things up. Go bowling, roller skating, dancing . . . #wycwyc

* Choose the stairs, every chance you get. #wycwyc

* Pace or go for a walk every time you're on the phone. Your butt is not glued to your office chair. #wycwyc

* Commercial break? Lunge around the TV room. Hold a squat. Have a tree pose contest. #wycwyc

* Use a rake instead of a leaf blower. Burn calories, clean the yard, save the air. #wycwyc

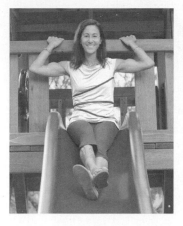
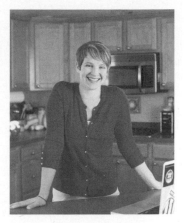

ABOUT THE AUTHORS

• •

CARLA BIRNBERG

Carla Birnberg's health philosophy (and life motto) is "Fitness isn't about fitting in." She believes we may all share the goal of a longer, healthier, more vibrant life, yet it's okay—even encouraged—to carve a unique path. Her site's tagline, "unapologetically myself," has inspired thousands to pursue goals in their own ways. Carla launched a popular blog called MizFitOnline in 2007, where she shared health and fitness knowledge with humor and ease. She quickly became known for jettisoning gym workouts in favor of "PLAYouts" with her daughter. She has since expanded her site, now at CarlaBirnberg.com, to cover everything from personal development to motherhood. Carla's engaging, keep-it-real advice has been featured in *Runner's World, Women's Day, The Wall Street Journal, Fitness, Ladies Home Journal, Glamour, Women's Health, Better Homes and Gardens,* Shape.com, and more. Carla is one of the major fitness brands' favorite voices: Carla was named one of Athleta's Five Favorite Fitness Blogs, and she was chosen a Transform Your Workout Fitness Expert by Café Mom. *Shape* magazine placed her in the Top Five Fitness Blogs, as well as One of 15 Fitness Gurus You Need To Follow On Twitter. She became Fila brand's inaugural spokesmom, and is a consultant to Venus Williams, who identified her as a social media influencer. You can find her online at CarlaBirnberg.com and on Twitter at @carla_birnberg.

RONI NOONE

In 2005, Roni Noone started a blog to help her stay accountable while trying to lose weight. This wasn't the first time Roni dieted, but it ended up being her last! Roni used her blog, called *Roni's Weigh*, not only to shed 70 pounds but to start a running habit, get over a fear of weight training, complete two marathons, and run seven Tough Mudders (yes, seven!). Recognizing the power of blogging, Roni created a supportive online community called BlogToLose, where thousands of users are blogging to reach their own weight-loss goals. In 2010, Roni launched the FitBloggin' conference to bring together new and seasoned health and wellness, fitness, and weight-loss bloggers for knowledge, personal growth, and networking. Now in its sixth year, FitBloggin' is a thriving, supportive community of bloggers sharing the conference's mission to spread a culture of health and wellness. Roni has represented and consulted with a wide variety of clients in the health and fitness industry, including Kellogg, ALDI, The Laughing Cow, Reebok, New Balance, HumanaVitality, Weight Watchers, Kraft, Vitalicious, Subway, Johns Hopkins University, Quaker, Nutrilite, and Pom. She has also been featured in many media outlets, including CNN, the *Today* show, *Inside Edition, Ladies Home Journal, Everyday Health, Woman's World, Woman's Day,* and *Wired*. You can find her at RoniNoone.com and on Twitter at @RoniNoone.

SELECTED TITLES FROM SEAL PRESS

The Nonrunner's Marathon Guide for Women: Get Off Your Butt and On with Your Training, by Dawn Dais. $17.00, 978-1-58005-205-4. Cheer on your inner runner with this accessible, funny, and practical guide.

Yogalosophy: 28 Days to the Ultimate Mind-Body Makeover, by Mandy Ingber. $18.00, 978-1-58005-445-4. Celebrity yoga instructor Mandy Ingber offers a realistic, flexible, daily plan that will help readers transform their minds, their bodies, and their lives.

Better Than Perfect: 7 Strategies to Crush Your Inner Critic and Create a Life You Love, by Elizabeth Lombardo. $16.00, 978-1-58005-549-9. A proven, powerful method for shaking the chains of perfectionism and finding balance in life.

Toss the Gloss: Beauty Tips, Tricks & Truths for Women 50+, by Andrea Q. Robinson. $24.00, 978-1-58005-490-4. Industry insider Andrea Q. Robinson—former beauty editor at *Vogue,* president of Tom Ford Beauty, and more—shares her ultimate guide to looking great at age 50 and beyond.

The Good Mother Myth: Redefining Motherhood to Fit Reality, edited by Avital Norman Nathman. $16.00, 978-1-58005-502-4. This collection of essays takes a realistic look at motherhood and provides a platform for real voices and raw stories, each offering an honest perspective on what it means to be a mother.

The 3-Day Reset: Restore Your Cravings for Healthy Foods in Three Easy, Empowering Days, by Pooja Mottl. $22.00, 978-1-58005-527-7. These 10 simple resets target and revamp your eating habits in practical, three-day increments.

FIND SEAL PRESS ONLINE

www.sealpress.com
www.facebook.com/sealpress
Twitter: @SealPress